WILDCARD

Navigating OCD and Mood Disorders

Casey Birchman

Amazon Kindle Direct Publishing

This book is dedicated to all those who suffer from mental illness. May they soon find the path to inner peace.

CONTENTS

Title Page
Dedication
Chapter One — 1
Chapter Two — 14
Chapter Three — 28
Chapter Four — 43
Chapter Five — 61
Chapter Six — 80
Chapter Seven — 100
About The Author — 111

Crisis Lines in the U.S.

Suicide hotline: Call 988
Text GO to 741741 to text with a professional

All the names and program names in this book have been omitted or changed in order to keep the privacy of those involved.

CHAPTER ONE

Introduction

Hello there! This isn't your typical book so I thought I'd introduce myself. My name is Casey, and I'm in college studying East Asian Languages and Cultures and minoring in Teaching ESL. I like creative writing, track and field, anime, and animals. This is the true me.

I also have an extreme case of OCD and depression (regulated by therapy and meds). I have a history of self-harm, intermittent explosive disorder, and ADHD as well. This is also my true self.

But when it comes to describing yourself, which side do you choose? Or do you choose both? Both are valid parts of yourself and very real in the eyes of ourselves and everyone around us. For me, I try to harness each part of myself. the struggles and the joys. But try not to get lost in the struggles. Rule number one I learned throughout my years of struggle is: don't let your mental illness be the ONLY thing that defines you.

You define you.

I hope you read this book with that rule in mind as we venture into the darkest recesses of our brains; the parts we wish we could live without. I know that for most of you reading this, you are looking for answers, answers to why you do the things you do; why you feel certain things and how to carry on despite them. Others may be reading this because they want to better understand a loved one who suffers from OCD or a mood disorder. In this book, I try my very hardest to come up with anecdotes, advice, and information that I have gathered in my six long years of treatment and seven of suffering from the debilitating mental illnesses mentioned above.

There is no one right way to read this book. If you want to skim through most and skip to a section that interests you or you think will act as a guide to help you along in your treatment journey, go ahead, skip around as much as you'd like. I do, however, think there is a certain benefit one can get from reading the whole thing, as it not only gives tips and tricks but also tells my personal story. Sometimes it's joining along on the journey of someone's struggles and contextualizing everything that makes the tips and tricks all the more poignant and useful.

This may seem all too familiar for people who have experienced true fear as a result of their mental illness and will act as a place to start, or for those who are reading this for a loved one, or just to learn more about OCD and mood disorders. Do you know what it feels like to have the rug pulled out from under you? Yes, of course you do—everybody does. Each one of us is intimately familiar with that sharp intake of breath that proceeds the White Room of your mind reserved for your anxiety with a rush of frantic thoughts and emotions that cascade from the center of your chest. Why is this happening? What can I do to fix it? I'm stuck. How can I get this to stop, why is everything ruined, I can't believe it, what'll I do? And then, right when you think you can't take the thrashing of your overwhelming emotions, you come to a conclusion. A solution. I'll borrow money so I can pay rent next month. Relief. Stepping on a crack in the sidewalk probably won't be the straw that breaks my mom's back. Relief. I'm generally a good person, I won't end up in jail. Certainty. You breathe a sigh, if you can't trust anyone else to help guide your decisions, you can at least trust yourself. Right?

There is a select chunk of the population who, for some reason or another, will enter the White Room and never leave to be greeted by that sweet relief at the exit. Who, instead of being lucky enough to be granted the privilege of trusting their compass of morals or rational thought upon internal reflection, will reach inside themselves and pull out some cracked hunk of metal and glass with the needles twitching every which direction. For some, this sad excuse for a compass will have been slightly off from the beginning. For others, they never really looked closely enough to notice anything going wrong, and by the time they've entered the White Room one too many times, this thing they've been taught to utilize as a precious tool in their darkest hours has malfunctioned. It has broken with the kind of jumpy sad movements of a cat losing its senses close to death.

The White Room functions, funnily enough, as a blinding fluorescent trap amidst the dark inky black recesses of our minds. This is where fear resides as pale walls, which close to entrap your charged and vicious thoughts. This is not the place you go when you're worried about passing an exam or you worry about that race you're about to run. This is not a place which forgives lightly. The exits in the White Room are far and few, and without a functioning compass you WILL remain lost inside.

No, the White Room is the place you go when you stare Death in the face, when the shrieking in your head splinters and reverberates off the inside of your skull. When your heart races as the blood drips off your arm and stings under the shower water. Tiptoes on the edge of a building, convinced you are about to dive off and plunge into the very worst urges of your nature.

I have been to that place, and it's the closest I've felt to Hell.

This was a stop on my journey through OCD.

Aside from a heap of mental disorders that crept up like a vice in my family, we have a tenacious light that holds us together and brightens my childhood. As a hyper-imaginative twenty-four-year-old, I still often feel like I have more of a connection to childhood than I do to adulthood. I almost feel like a naive child who has been granted the ability to drink, drive, and sleep with whomever I choose. I suppose though, when I really think about it, there is a black somber distance between me and my child self.

CASEY BIRCHMAN

When I look back on the person I once was, before the White Room, I see a golden light, almost too beautiful to be true, ringing with nostalgia that touches every aspect of *my younger self* ...

Innocent beginnings

The first time I realized I could have OCD was in my AP psychology class senior year of high school. Mrs. S showed us a video of people ritualizing and I gasped.

"That's literally me! That's exactly what I do!" I said to my friend who smiled and cocked his head.

"Huh. Really?"

OCD is a genetic illness, but that doesn't mean there aren't certain features to one's life that shape the way one's brain is formed towards those tendencies. I consider my childhood to be perfect. A perfect little fairytale swathed in shimmering golden light. But there were telltale signs of my illness early on. While I thought they were just quirks at the time or me presenting as a worry wart big sibling, the ways which I perceived my world started shaping up the perfect storm when I was eighteen:

Mom laughed at us in the sunlight as swallows swooped daringly around our heads and back under the pier. I shot down to avoid the bird and accidentally stepped on a slimy rock on the floor of the water. I screeched and kicked furiously back towards the raft where my cousins played.

"Dum-Dum! I stepped on Dum-Dum!" I yelled with a tone of playfulness in my voice and real fear in my eyes.

"What do you mean, Dum-Dum? Is it really there?" My cousin Percy giggled in confusion.

"It's this ancient rock. It's just—just this freaky *thing*."

"Casey, what?" Mom laughed incredulously and we kept on playing.

Dum-Dum. I first met Dum-Dum a few years back in that magnificent movie *Night at the Museum*. He was the Easter Island head that came to life every night along with the rest of the displays and artifacts when the museum closed on account of an ancient Egyptian tablet. His catchphrase "Dum-Dum want gum gum" made him stick with me. I could feel the smooth ridges of his rock face; his grey jaws pushing the giant ball of gum in his stone mouth. His surface was cool. It would feel wonderful to chomp into that gum. Or his face. He was an alluring mystery, which was a perfect match for my underwater enemy, the slimy rock.

An important distinction to make, it's not that I actually *thought* there was an ancient Easter Island head resting beneath the surface of the water, but it's that I *felt* there was. My visceral imagination had locked onto the shape, the feel, the lore of this giant CGI Easter Island head and filled in the blanks when I felt something I couldn't otherwise see under the water. It's also important to realize that my perception of reality overruled anyone else's, and that while I could fully believe it was there in my heart, in the distant corners of my mind I knew it was only a regular old rock.

Mom wouldn't ever come in contact with Dum-Dum though, she'd just sit near us on the pier and watch over us like the swallows protecting their nests, making sure none of us drowned. Xavier didn't know how to swim, so he wore a life vest.

Another important thing to know about me is that my brain likes to latch onto sensations. Oh and it just loooveess similes and metaphors. Eats those up for breakfast. The water was pudding without my glasses on; it pushed me up—I was flying with the fish, but it was also thick and dense enough to hold up a boat. This hyper-imaginative brain of mine played into an important part of my intrusive thoughts, images, and urges when I got older.

Xavier didn't know how to swim. The inky smoothness of the water caressing my body—you can drink, fly, and throw—allowed me to play for hours. "Be careful guys! Don't hit your head on the pier." Tight fear. **Xavier didn't know how to swim.** I stayed with one hand on Xavier's raft the rest of the day.

Scenes like these would turn out to be the beginnings of my worried thought patterns which lead to my horrible OCD later on in life. It was nobody's fault, it was just that I felt like I had to watch out for my brother and the possibility of him drowning even with a life vest on seemed so great, that it struck me to my core.

At first, the qualities of OCD that I had seemed to make me a good, responsible person. Or a quirky one depending on the obsessions and rituals people witnessed. But these were actually warning signs everybody, including myself, missed which led to my downfall in 2016.

But what is OCD?

For anyone who doesn't realize it, OCD is a complicated and tricky bastard of an illness. It is formed out of good intentions that warp until it literally drives you mad. If the definition of insanity is doing the same thing over and over again to try and get different results, then people with OCD are most definitely plagued with a sort of insanity. That, I can agree with because for people who have suffered with severe OCD such as myself, life becomes a living hell; every moment is torture—you may not even get relief in sleep either because you can't fall asleep or because your fears haunt your dreams (as if you weren't already living your worst nightmare).

OCD can be many things and have many faces. It can show in the form of physical or mental compulsions and can be something as unnoticeable as picturing something specific to counter an intrusive thought to loudly making an extra sound after you hear a certain word spoken. Some of my rituals consisted of: cutting my tongue on my retainer repetitively, wearing mismatching socks, saying "cow" in my head after I had an unpleasant thought, imagining fish in my mouth, extreme over cleaning, wiping so hard it drew blood, clicking my heels together a certain way, rewriting letters and numbers, researching, rereading, checking my surroundings and body constantly for abnormalities, avoiding bad luck, warning others of things I thought to be dangerous, and many many more things that must have seemed extremely odd to an outside viewer.

OCD is the stickiest mental illness I know of. Stingers in the form of hooks stab and grab at thoughts until they are transformed into fears, and those fears stick to more thoughts until it's a completely tangled hivemind. Overwhelming and overbearing. One thought becomes another until you have so many you try desperately to remember each one somehow so you can best protect yourself and the people around you.

When I was deathly afraid my cats might die from lily

toxicity, I got into a car accident because I was typing notes that I "had" to remember on my phone. It punctured the front of my car and the airbag went off, bruising and burning my left arm and leaving me in shock. The guy in front of me hit and bruised his head on the steering wheel and oh boy was he angry. I think about that moment a lot: I was so wrapped up in my own little world and so worried about hurting my pets that I hurt other people and myself in the process.

That's what happened to my favorite plant I had from fifth grade to freshman year of college. And my friends betta fish. And my old dog April. Those fish and that plant died because I smothered them with worried love, and I tripped over my dog lunging to grab her because I was freaking out the moment I let her leash go by accident. She ended up having scars. OCD can be so extreme that you end up paying for your worry in big, tangible ways. Your life isn't just destroyed by thoughts, it's destroyed by your actions.

Here we come to the cognitive triad. Thoughts, feelings, and actions make up each side. The only thing you can control, and therefore, change are your actions/behaviors. And since each side is connected, each side in turn becomes affected by the changes in your actions.

The action side for someone suffering from an untreated case of OCD is made up of rituals or compulsions. As people with OCD know, these types of rituals are not just doing a cutesy little luck ritual for a baseball game, these can literally take up every waking hour of your life. You may spend an hour turning the light switch on and off and shaking your head while grunting because the way you've done it doesn't seem "right," and you feel as if something bad is going to happen if you can't get the right experience that comes with the actions. You may not be able to eat because you are so busy going over mental lists in your head to try and ward off the excruciating fear that you have forgotten something, and that someone will come to serious harm if you don't remember it.

The way I try to explain the motivation to perform rituals

to a person without OCD is this: imagine you have this pet peeve that makes you feel anxious if you don't fix it or do away with it. Let's say someone leaves the drawers open. At first you just go around shutting them because it makes the kitchen look untidy, and then it becomes a habit. Sometimes you open a drawer and then shut it yourself, just to feel the satisfaction of completing the action. It feels soothing, right in some way you can't explain. The next time you see a drawer that has been left open you feel a rush of anxiety because it isn't how you are used to things being, it just feels *wrong* in some way, like you can't move on from the kitchen until you've shut that drawer, and shutting it feels so satisfying. It takes your anxiety away and you can now move on to doing other things ... unless maybe you need to open it and close it a few more times until it feels like the anxiety has really gone away or until you feel better about it. This is for many people how rituals get started. I know for me this is how many of my less overbearing rituals started forming in early childhood, like shaking a bottle of green dye every night once on the left, then once on the right, and then once hard in the middle. I had to do this until I felt and thought the "right" thought every single night before I could fall asleep. If I didn't, I believed I would have bad luck the next day, and I would be too anxious to fall asleep. It's little seemingly "quirky" rituals you have to be aware of when they first show up so you can nip them in the bud before they blossom into the tangle of weeds that is a major case of OCD. Once you've waited too long, things will have probably taken over your life, and you will end up where some of you may be: in some sort of treatment center.

    OCD and anxiety are like your mind's broken alarm systems. I feel badly for them because the hidden truth is their anxiety and rituals are actually ways that your brain is trying to help you; to save you. It's not like the boy who cried wolf, because to anxiety, there actually *is* a problem to be seen and dealt with. It is an overreaction however, one that can leave you wrung out and flailing. One that takes over your life until there is no interval of peace in between the blaring alarms. Your brain has the natural tendency to want to protect you from danger. With OCD, it's just like everything is a danger—everything that corresponds with your values that is.

OCD and anxiety are not just alarm systems, they're also beacons of your values. The way they shed light on your values is this: if you are worried about something happening, you know that the thing it affects is something you hold dear to you. For example, I thought I knew that people close to me were going to die. Instead of that meaning they are in imminent danger like OCD makes you believe, it actually just means that you care deeply about them; enough that everything around you starts to seem like a major threat.

The summer of 2019, when I was at my absolute worst levels of anxiety, panic, and rituals in my life, I didn't just think that my cats were going to die, I *knew* it to be true. I knew their lives were in imminent danger every day. I left the house without doing rituals because there were lilies (that are toxic to cats) everywhere in our neighborhood.

I couldn't sleep, couldn't eat— I lost ten pounds in 10 days. I vomited multiple times a day which was basically just stomach bile because I was so overcome with anxiety. I thought there was lily pollen everywhere in the house, and that to be safe, I had to do a number of rituals that took all day and night, constant round the clock work to keep up with. When one ritual would be done, it would give me such a fleeting sense of relief that I almost wouldn't even feel it before moving onto the next one. NOTHING was enough. **Nothing will ever be enough for OCD**. I vacuumed the basement, but each time I would step backwards, I would step on contaminated carpet meaning I was just retracking "all of the lily pollen" around after I did so. I had walked into the basement bathroom after coming in from outside before I vacuumed, but then I had to use it, and before I took my socks off, I stepped outside of the room tracking even more in. Oops, that meant I had to vacuum again, but then the vacuum broke and it turns out, it was just spitting out what I had sucked in the entire time so then the pollen must be all over the place. That means you have to lock the cats out of the basement and move their food and litter upstairs, but I wasn't done with rituals upstairs so I had to move them into Xavier's room which is small and heats up tremendously at night.

I would go in there to give them fresh water, but in the process, I track in pollen everytime, meaning I have to vacuum without letting them escape and pick all the crunched up leaves that I just *know* are lily leaves. But that just doesn't take the fear away, doesn't leave my OCD satisfied so then I have to stay up all night taking them in three different rooms, trying to roll them off and torturing them by picking them up and wiping them off and using a lint roller on them, which they are afraid of and makes them uncomfortable. Then once I finally think I've done all I can do for the night and I just may need sleep to function, I see what appears to be a chocolate stain on the carpet of Alexa's room, and I have to work late into the hours of the morning, switching rooms once again.

The pull of a compulsion to a person with OCD is extremely strong. It feels like if you don't complete it, all of your worst fears will become stunningly real, all in technicolor. I'm here to tell you that that becomes *better*. With treatment (ERP), you CAN and WILL get better at resisting compulsions. And the drive to do many of them will be lessened or even eradicated all together!

ERP, or exposure and response prevention, is a technique that involves making a list of your triggers and fears in a hierarchy with a licensed therapist, then creating personalized challenges that will make you anxious. You must allow the anxiety to be there while you sit with it. Any attempts you make to get rid of it nullifies the exposure. So you're sitting in brutal hell with this exposure and then you begin to notice something as the clock "tick tick ticks" along. Your anxiety is going down. You feel less anxious at the end of this than you did at the start and that, my friend, is a feeling of relief, real relief, not the false relief that rituals give you.

Usually, while your anxiety may go down doing ERP, the trigger you are working on may never completely go away as something that bothers you. The main point is, anxiety does not equal pain or danger, but instead, it equals discomfort; something that through therapy, you can learn to sit with and deal with in day-to-day life. The process of learning that by rewiring your brain is as hard as it is intense. There may be crying, frustration, anger, but the reward of being free from OCD's thorny grasp is overpowering and shines out against all of those things.

CHAPTER TWO

The Downfall

Sometimes OCD can rear its ugly head at the most inopportune times—in fact, it usually does. There's never really a good time for a trigger or a compulsion to pop up. One of the first times I had a major, and I mean *major*, trigger pop up, I was innocently in school, not yet realizing that my world was going to change. For those of you who don't know, it can be as simple as that, one thought can send a person into a frenzy, a whirlwind of something feral even though one minute ago they seemed completely fine …

Daydreaming at my desk, a beloved pastime of mine, I would prop my head up on my hand and listen with one ear while my mind was wrapped in excitement. Action sequences would play out across fields of rough terrain. What if Zero from *Vampire Knight* was alive? Would I be friends with him at school? A frog hopped across the front of my mind trailing a line of flags behind it. Blue red green purple red. Red. Iron Man is red; I love him. What if Tony and Steve got together? I wondered idly if my sister Alexa thought either was cute. I wrinkled my nose, reeling. *Tony's mine to cherish and protect and bond with.* Alexa's name is red. Steve and Tony should be together, they were already close. It would be hot; love is red too. What if Steve could only be thrust into this world with the help of someone else's soul? And of course he'd need a body …

A rope snapped and I was shoved into sticky red quicksand as I suddenly came up with a scenario that would haunt me for months: if Captain America came to life and his mind was put into a new attractive body of a stranger, but part of Alexa's mind was mixed in with his, and I fell in love with him without knowing she was in there, when I found out, would I stay in love? Red behind my eyes, everything was bright hot red bearing down on my conscience. Tony's suit was red like love, like Alexa and suddenly, as they describe it in the novelizations, a coffin—I was, for the first time, entrapped by a thing supposed to protect me.

Tony loved Steve and I loved Steve ... and Alexa? In what way? Do I have a crush on her right now? The red seeped into the marrow of my bones. I was contaminated. I felt itchy and dirty and everything was wrong. I was growing more uncomfortable in my own skin by the second. I wanted to tear it off. I would if that meant getting away from this rancid feeling.

I had to be in love with her, otherwise why would this thought keep sticking? I had to accept that in some capacity I was in love with her, or at least I *could* fall in love with her, and wasn't that just as bad as being in love with your own sister currently? *I want to commit incest, I'm a rapist.* The thought pounded in my head for weeks. No matter how many forcefields and sacred cows (mental rituals) I pushed into the forefront of my mind to fight, the thought could not be defeated. I recall sitting on stage at graduation just reeling and repeating and repeating and repeatingandrepeatingandrepeatingrepeatingrepeatingrepeating , shaking my head to clear myself of the thoughts, tears welling in my eyes. My family took me out to dinner at my favorite restaurant. The waiter took our picture. The smile did not reach my eyes.

Alexa, of course, came with us on our yearly vacation to South Carolina soon after graduation, and the pretty scenery did nothing to quiet the thoughts. In fact, now with more time on my hands, the barrage of thoughts just became louder and more and more convincing. I remember sitting in the car on the sixteen hour drive, my headphones plugged in as I tried desperately to drown out the noise of my thoughts, the weight of their connotations, over and over and over and over. It was maddening. When after hours I finally realized distractions wouldn't work, I tried reasoning with the thoughts; coming up with new scenarios in which I wouldn't be in love with this Steve-Alexa hybrid thing.

I engaged in what I would come to know were extreme checking behaviors. I would play out a fictional scenario in my head, like me hugging Steve, or helping him get used to the world after he had just sprung forth from the comics and then I would A. see how the scene ended, B. make sure my heart had no attraction to his own, and C. make sure there were no visceral responses my body would react with as I thought of the increasingly steamy scenarios. I did this even after we arrived. Pausing my music in order to think hard enough about the scenario, in order to "solve" it, to come out at the end of my imaginary scenario convinced there was no way I could ever develop feelings for the hybrid.

The rituals and obsessions became worse and worse and didn't stop for anything anyway even after I came to that conclusion because it turned out that was just reassurance, which for people with OCD goes away fleetingly. I remember sitting there in an almost catatonic state, trying desperately to get these images and thoughts out of my head. That only made it worse of course, but I didn't have any tools to help myself at that point.

Around ten o'clock, my cousins and siblings jumped in the glowing pool with the multicolored lights. "Where's Casey?" I heard my cousin Lyle call out into the muggy night.

"I think they went back inside." A loud splash and a shrill scream.

"Aww how come?" Xavier touted. I shut the door as quietly as I could.

"Because they're an idiot!" Lyle cried.

My heart cracked a hairline fracture that had always been absent when I was called names. Names we siblings and cousins called each other didn't ever mean anything, but something about this time made my toes curl with disgust. My heart beat in my ears red-hot with shame. I just couldn't stand to be in the pool with Alexa, with any of them. In swimsuits leaping around. Reminding me that one day someone would look at each of them in longing. What if that person would be me? Have I already become an incestuous pedophile?

"Hey Case-o! Already old and tired like the rest of us?" Gramp asked when I came back inside. I shrugged, hair dripping shower water onto my pajamas, and plastered on a small grin.

"Yeah, I just wanted to—" *What if Steve's hair looked this way in the breeze? Then there's no way I wouldn't start to fall in love with him? I guess I could just say to myself that I'm ignoring the sister part of him but doesn't that still make me a pedophile—*

"You alright there Casey?"

My breathing accelerated. I could feel my heartbeat pound in my chest. I rubbed my fingers together at my sides. I faked a yawn.

"I dunno, I'm seriously tired, lol." I turned and walked upstairs toward my room. *What if they could tell?*

"Good night!"

"Night," I said flatly with tears in my eyes. *Do they know they're living with a disgusting criminal while they call me nicknames and give me hugs?* I felt queasy. No snack for me I guess.

I awoke to the array of sound of the television blaring and what sounded like a few of the other kids screaming in the pool, and in that blessed instant, I wasn't tormented by the thoughts. For a fuzzy moment suspended away from the rest of time, I was calm, at peace, the rest of the world in front of me. Images of the beach flashed in front of my eyes, and I could feel a shot of excitement. That woke me up. Thrust me back into a sick reality that only sleep could provide a break from. *Steve would be ripped! And wet from the water. He'd be turned on and if he liked me ... what if I knew in the first place that she was in there too? Would I still be attracted to him, oh god!*

I tiptoed up to my parents' room to find that it was already empty. I guess that I slept in much longer than I'd previously thought. The sink was running.

"Mom?" I called out cautiously.

"Yeah?" I came in as she left the bathroom and immediately started shaking and crying. "Sweetie! What is going on?!"

"I can't tell you!!" I sobbed in shame. Here I was, the

blackest of black souls finally breaking and seeking comfort in my innocent unassuming mother. I, in no way, deserved her generosity and kindness, and yet I took it willingly. That made me even worse of a person.

I wet her shoulder as she held me and rubbed my back. I felt the quills on my back stabbing her and shooting out poison that seeped into her skin. I was the definition of evil. I was a sludge beast that silently infiltrated and contaminated everything she touched. I cried even harder.

"Tell me what on earth is wrong honey," she said in her joking tone.

"What would you do … if you thought you were in love with someone and it turned out to be your brother?"

"What?" she laughed. "Hon*ey*! That's ridiculous. How would I not have known from the start?" I stomped and growled, surprising both of us. My voice became higher and coarser, and I all but shrieked quietly as I went on, becoming increasingly frustrated, unable to contain myself any longer.

"No, like, if for some reason there was this magic disguise and then they turned out to be Uncle James or something? Would you still be in love with him?"

"Honey, that's gross."

I cried out and ripped myself away from her loving grasp, then stomped back to my room and slammed the door shut.

"Nevermind!" I yelled, locking it. There are no words to describe the amount of fury, shame, guilt, and sadness that wracked my body at that moment. It was red, bright blood red splattering on the wall on the sheets turning black and oozing through everything the spatters touched. I clenched my fists so hard that my fingernails cut my palms. I tested the limits of my anger. First I stomped. I didn't feel better, in a "I feel sort of better" way. It was addictive: the split second outlet it gave.

A violent need shot through my arm, and I hit the desk. A jolt of power like I hadn't felt since I was very little. I threw the pillows around, slapped the bedsheet, kicked the door. I felt high with a reddish pinkish blackish hue that I had never felt in this extreme before. Making little squeaking sounds, I fell into the bathroom, mind still through all of this laughing at me, trying to force me to solve the Steve scenario. I needed it OUT!

"I never want to think about this again!" I bit out in a high rumble as I suddenly stepped forward. I'd ripped the towel rack clean out of the wall.

I stood there panting, plaster covering my hands, and just stared and looked at them. I could feel my face going white and for one moment I was free: something else took priority of thought and slapped the thought out of my head. I learned right then and there, the only way to get rid of a damning thought was to force it out—a realization I later learned was totally and utterly incorrect.

The right way, I learned later that year, was to allow thoughts to come and to sit with the huge amount of anxiety that comes with it. Only then could it start to fade away ...

This continual cloud cover that overtakes your mind is typical of OCD. And when people start obsessing over something others don't understand, it can be extremely frustrating. And this can lead to anger outbursts and rapid changes in mood.

Another thing that goes side by side with intrusive thoughts but isn't talked about as much are intrusive urges. These urges are only superficial, not what someone really wants at their core, but they pester them, nonetheless. For me, these came in the form thinking I wanted to grab my sister or slap her or even kiss her, and with each added new fear and obsession, they changed and grew in intensity because I tried my hardest to block them out instead of letting them exist without acting on them (which I will get into more detail about later).

Tips and Tricks for Dealing With OCD

- Lean into the possibility that what's feared may happen (this may mean telling yourself that it WILL happen and sitting with it.
- Do ERP (exposure and response prevention. I will go into that in more detail later on).
- Any mood can breed OCD, but especially stress AND eustress.
- You can be upset about it another day.
- Don't feel badly if you find yourself purposely triggering yourself not for the exposure. Your brain may be used to chewing on something or you're used to feeling agitated and upset.
- Do what scares you every day.
- OCD treatment is a lifestyle, it never ends. This is a GOOD thing, keeping up with treatment in your head gets easier and easier overtime, much better than having to go back to a treatment center or intensive therapy. You may find yourself only doing little things to keep your OCD in check, or a bigger trigger may pop up and you'll have to pull out the big guns. (Usually there will be smaller things though.)
- Don't rely on others to tell you what is and isn't how to handle your OCD. Listen to your therapist and rely on your own tool set. Ex: your friend says that calling the vet and double-checking something is completely rational because they do it too. NO, you have OCD, you have to live your life differently.
- Reinforce your support system with friends and family who have talked with your therapist and who actually know the correct aspects of OCD treatment.
- You're allowed to get frustrated! Keeping up with OCD is draining and difficult. Just don't let your frustration get you off track.

- DON'T GIVE INTO COMPULSIONS, no matter how tempting they may be. OCD is an extremely slippery slope.
- Be open with your friends and family about your mental illnesses.
- Connect with people who suffer the same diagnosis as you (even though they may be on different points in their journey, you can still find comfort in learning someone has the same thoughts or compulsions as you).
- Join the conversation! Educate people about OCD. Crush the stereotypes!
- Relapses are normal. Progress is never a straight line. It's like some kid scribbled all over a graph.
- Treatment takes TIME and absolute A+ EFFORT to be completely effective. Don't slack off! If you want to be free in the future, you've got to be willing to keep up with the dirty work, sometimes plunging into it.
- Some people will just never understand. And that's okay, remind yourself that you are still valid and loved all the same.
- What truly is a "bad" or "good" person? I'll let you think about that. PS, the answer is we are all good and bad because we have all done good and bad things.
- Nobody is perfect!
- Often the last thing we think is what we really feel, not necessarily the first.
- Some things get easier—but some things never get easier; you keep on fighting the fight anyway for your own soul to shine bright.
- Working out WILL make you feel emotionally better! It gives your mind and body something to chew on and provides relief on depression, too.
- Every brain has weird quirks that we may never totally understand. This could be OCD or how you think about thoughts or anything.

- The point isn't to get rid of urges to ritualize, it's to sit with them because sometimes you won't be able to get rid of them.
- When we imagine things, it gets extreme and out of hand zippity quick. And seems so real and free in your head, clearing it seems more possible.
- Different people think about death differently.
- It's okay to be okay with how you think.
- Think about it—not all OCD fears are the same; one person could totally not understand or be trapped by another person's fears. Hmm …
- Sometimes you can make a bizarre connection and have an intrusive thought by thinking of two conflicting things, but somehow, one reminds you of another and "contaminates" it. This can be a color in the back of your mind, a certain body position or feeling, or who knows what else connects them. That's the connection. Nothing inherently gross or bad about the second thing exists.
- Rituals and obsessions can be anything! Nothing is too weird for OCD.
- Make a body checker sheet to check in with how you are feeling. Draw or print an outline of a body and use colored markers to draw where you feel your emotions. Have a list of questions ready: What am I feeling? Where am I feeling it? Is there anything I need? On a scale of one to ten how anxious am I? If you are at a ten, have a list of coping skills, and circle a few you'd like to try. For lower level anxiety, have a list of tools you can use to sit with the anxiety (resist compulsions, do exposures, etc.).

Obsessions I've Had:

- Tongue falling apart
- Heart attack
- Something under my bed
- Killing my pets brutally
- Killing my family
- Raping children
- Serotonin syndrome
- Killing old people
- People slipping or tripping (esp. Old people)
- Having sex with my family
- Pushing someone onto the train tracks
- Worried about poisoning pets (lily pollen, grapes, chocolate, etc.)
- Tapeworm/parasite, getting and passing one
- Best friend dying in a car crash
- Cancer
- Brain tumor
- Neurological problem
- Worrying if I told someone to kill themselves online
- Second guessing self
- Ferret cage not closed
- Gas leak
- Stove on
- Carbon monoxide
- Friends dying
- Other loved ones dying
- Pets dying
- Bleeding internally
- Slitting my throat if I looked at a knife too long
- Kicking kittens because it was "cool" to some people so it might be cool to me
- Molesting my pets
- Attacking people I'm jealous of

- Crushing baby birds
- Dropping babies
- Thinking I was going blind
- Thinking I was hallucinating (when I wasn't)
- Thinking I had schizophrenia
- Thinking my skin would fall off
- Getting a hernia
- Having colon cancer
- Having stomach cancer
- One of my organs exploding
- Falling off a cliff
- Getting trapped in the middle of nowhere
- Someone's car exploding in front of me
- Pinworms
- Getting shit on things outside of the bathroom
- Peeing my pants
- Thinking our car would explode
- Thinking spiders would bite me
- Thinking I'll get DID (dissociative identity disorder)
- Choking on pills
- Accidental overdose
- Accidental mixing of meds or alcohol
- Family dying if didn't do a ritual
- Bloodborne illness
- STI
- Falling in love with someone evil
- Accidentally carrying a firearm or bomb in the airport when I have no access to such items
- Falling off a balcony
- Pets falling out the window
- Thinking people could read my thoughts (intrusive thoughts—thoughts can't be sent off into the world; they just bounce against the inside of your skull. Try it and see what happens. You can wish something or have hope, but the simple state of wishing or hoping doesn't do anything to further your goal—actions do.)

And many many more ...

Intentional Thinking

Sometimes you find yourself drowning in repetitive thoughts. Something jerks you out of your sleepy life, and you are jarringly, glaringly, acutely aware of something and how disturbing or disgustingly repulsive it is, and OCD's claws unhook and snag it so tight that even rigorous therapy won't let you forget it. This doesn't mean the anxiety or disgust or triggered emotions won't completely go away, it just means it's a thought you have more than most people, and you can notice it gently. One of the things we learned in program was the story of the unwelcome party guest. In this story, you are invited to a party and you have three choices: you can stay at home and miss out on all the fun because you're worried about something, let's say some intrusive thoughts. You could also go to the party and engage with the guest, who riled you up like no other and takes away the fun, and then you're wondering why you went in the first place. *Or* you can go and just acknowledge the guest is there; make small talk. Notice he is there, and do not engage. This way, you have the optimal partying experience. It's the same thing with intrusive thoughts.

For instance, I could be sitting in my car with a friend and suddenly realize they have genitals under their clothes; that I do, that my parents and children, who I have interacted with in my life, do too. I'm now picturing the genitals of each and every person who I just named. I feel like they are in my mouth or I'll do or say something inappropriate to my peer in the car or I'll creep them out. Now I can do a few different things with this. I can either:

A. Wonder why I'm thinking about this in the first place and decide what kind of fucked up person this makes me and dwell on it so much the images and sensations and judgement pile up and pound away at my sense of peace,

B. I can avoid them by doing rituals, mental or physical, causing them to be more graphic and pronounced,

C. Purposely think more about the images, or

D. Just acknowledge they are thoughts that pop up in my head.

Both C and D are proper responses. You may ask yourself why C would be a proper response or how it could do absolutely anything to help the situation. Isn't that the opposite of what you want? To think about the spine tingling, vomit-inducing hell more? Well yes, because if you find yourself avoiding the images and thoughts, your OCD will do this fun little game that all of your siblings or cousins have done to you at some point which is called "when you stay and try to block them out or give them a heated response, they actually pester you more and more until you absolutely can't stand it." If you intentionally think the thoughts for the purpose of exposure, you will feel an increase in anxiety at first because you are facing the fear, but after doing it for a while, OCD loses interest, because you aren't giving it the response it wants to best pester you with.

While I know intrusive thoughts come from my own mind, they are not actually consistent with my core beliefs. This is why I made the voice of my intrusive thoughts a demon named Devon. Whenever I get anything from a bigoted intrusive thought on the bus, to a violent massacre pictured in my mind, I say, "Jeez Devon, chill" and laugh to myself. I try to acknowledge it is just Devon trying to bully me, and in a way, reminding me of my values and move on. Because my reaction is that I dislike my intrusive thoughts, I know they are the opposite to my values. Sometimes though, you may feel neutral about a thought or even lean into thinking it, this makes it harder to differentiate it from a normal, core belief thought, but with a therapist, you can parse it out as such.

CHAPTER THREE

The Worst It's Been

Sometimes a fear takes the shape of a ghost of a loved one. In my case, the death of my granny devastated me to the core. It was the first death in my life that seemed real to me, and yet there I sat, on the couch at her house, feeling as unreal as ever in my own body.

Large amounts of distress or stress can allow OCD to take hold, and this was it, my breaking point leading me to three more treatment centers for the next half year. And I didn't even care as I slipped and relapsed so hard I felt like I was the one who was going to end up dead. The thing is though, I became stupendously terrified that my pets would die. It all started when my dog ate a grape flavored meatball. (Yes they exist and they are really quite good.) But grapes are toxic to dogs. When my dad wouldn't take her to the vet, that left me shaken. What if she had died too?

We brought home lilies from my granny's memorial service. My anxiety immediately went into overdrive: Are lilies toxic to dogs, is this other flower? They are toxic to cats according to the vet. I checked and researched and asked for reassurance for the entire six-hour drive of hell back to my house. And then, outside, just as I had reached my safe home, death lined the sidewalks. I had learned enough about flowers on my trip down the rabbit hole and there were lilies in my own yard, and I had two cats that I loved from the bottom of my heart who were in my mind, in extreme immediate danger, even though they lived inside.

A few weeks after that doomed car ride, I found myself on my porch lost and alone in my obsessions that had completely taken over my life. I was doing rituals day in and day out which had taken a grave toll on my body and mind.

It was a gorgeous day, and death was blooming just a few feet away from me. The smell of hot wood and flowers overwhelmed me as I squeaked into the phone, desperately trying not to wake my mom who was sleeping inside. I wasn't crying: I don't think there were enough tears left in me at that point. I never took my focus off of those flowers as I paced on the porch running a hand through my sweaty hair.

"I think Huck is going to eat something. I know a piece of a lily was tracked inside by one of us by accident!" Salem, my best friend's mom's calm and measured voice sounded on the other end of the line beginning with a light "mhm."

"Well you know sweetie I don't think that that's even a big enough piece to be able to hurt him." Logic, for a split sweet second, seemed to ring true. But in my foolishness, I didn't think myself a fool, so I hissed back at her in desperation.

"No, I know what I saw and only one flake of pollen is enough to kill them!"

"Mmm, but honey you've been going in and out of that house for years and nothing bad has ever happened to either of them; I think it's gone by now right?"

Nausea rose in my stomach, rising over the hunger pains. I hadn't eaten anything in two days and had hardly anything to drink

"No, no. If I don't find it he'll never be safe! I can't!"

"Okaay, calm down. Take a deep breath and let's think through this okay?" I grunted in frustration and stomped down hard on the porch, immediately whipping my head to the door, afraid that I had awoken my mom who was sleeping peacefully inside.

"NO! No. I have to go inside and check on them again. I'm sorry ... I know this is really repetitive and stressful ... I'm freaking out! I can't stop! I can't eat, I can't sleep ..."

"I know honey, I know. Things are tough right now." I squeezed my free hand into a fist. I could feel myself shaking.

Apparently I did have room for more tears because they welled up in my eyes yet again and spilled onto the porch.

If someone walking outside saw me like this, I wouldn't have even cared. The safety of my cats was that important, my number one priority. And if I didn't do everything the most direct way to protect them, then I was doing them a disservice. More than that, I was leading them directly to their graves.

But the thought of waking my mom ... I didn't want to annoy her anymore than I had. Couldn't take the pity, the love I thought I didn't deserve as I wasn't protecting my pets. The panic was mounting at this point along with the nausea. I cried even harder struggling for words as my shame grew, knowing my best friend's mother had to listen to this over the phone.

"I'm sorry!" I cried out and then promptly vomited over the side of the porch. It wasn't the kind of vomit that leaves you feeling better afterwards, I struggled through it as it wracked my body, spewing up tiny flecks of food. I guess I had eaten something. When was that?

"Deep breaths honey. Why don't I stop by before my doctor's appointment? You can just chill out or we can get something and try to eat or anything."

I nodded, not realizing she couldn't see this action over the phone but not caring in the moment as I struggled to regain my voice.

"Yeah." I whispered. "Thanks."

"How about I come in an hour? Does that work okay with you?"

"Yeah. Thank you." I hung up.

My face was hot and bright red from the tears and the summer sun, and my feet were that special disgusting kind of dirty from the porch and the rancid smell from the death buds flooded my nose. I stomped again in frustration, hands curling into claws. I struck my leg repeatedly, hard enough to leave a bruise. I hated the world for doing this to me. To my cats. Putting them in danger and me, of all people, in charge of their fates. And I hated myself for being like this because a tiny, miniscule speck in the back of my mind taunted me, a normal person wouldn't be reacting like this, and wouldn't be putting this heavy burden on their friends. Their best friend. Their best friend's *mom* at four in the fucking morning. I would have to remember to cut myself in punishment when I could take a breath away from the pink and white pixie stick powder that was anxiety clinging to my ribcage and poisoning my heart.

Back inside every fiber of my being was screaming at me in a white-hot rage to check on the cats, but I just couldn't get past the door. Every step that I took into their domain could possibly contaminate them and kill them. *Murderer.* My chest panged. *Murderer!* I slapped myself to will the thoughts away. They were the most safe locked away in that little room, even if they could still die in there too. I resorted to listening to Huck's cries through the door to ascertain his well being. Well, that he was at least alive in there anyway, if not suffering from being enclosed in such a small area.

Next I tried to eat a few bites of a bagel and drink some water. My throat felt like it wouldn't let me swallow; like doing so would land a bomb in my intestines and corrupt me, prevent me from taking care of the cats. *My* cats. Who relied on me.

An hour passed in a hurry and Salem arrived right on time, pulling up without any fanfare outside of the house. I cleaned my feet off several times before finally slipping on my gym shoes and heading outside, concentrating hard to not step on possible lily hotspots in the grass near her car. I climbed into the passenger seat and let out all of my frustrations. My struggles and woes in a few sentences. She had a ginger ale for my stomach and had brought her knitting along. I was too afraid to leave the house and too sickly to feel like going anywhere, so she turned off her car, rolled down the windows, and let the morning air in as I sat straight up against the seat, one hand clasped around my phone and the other in my lap.

"I'm so tired ..." I croaked.

"You can rest here. Do whatever you need." Then there was nothing more to say and she pulled out her knitting, and for the first time in weeks, I took a breath and closed my eyes. I never really fell into a full sleep as I could hear the carbonation popping in the ginger ale and the click click clicking of Salem's knitting needles. But for the first time in such a long time, I felt the blissful release of rest overtake me as I sat there in the sunshine.

I felt safe with someone who I had grown up with, who wasn't possessed by madness. Who had created my best friend. I felt the tug of sleep pull at me for who knows how long and finally, finally I felt the fuzziness and grey and red chaos that was my mind blur out so it was almost see-through: it was as grey as her car seats. I was my own head, my own thoughts, my own beating heart and soul as I sat there fading in and out. It was the closest I felt to freedom.

There are lots of things that I did in this short piece I can now resist or identify as maladaptive. For starters, things as basic as eating and sleeping are monumental in helping ease the torture of any mental illness. When you don't sleep, your body is running on empty. Things get blown out of proportion and everything seems ten times more overwhelming. Soon after that day, I started hallucinating from lack of sleep, and that never helps anybody. Lack of eating is also a massive thing that many people don't even realize is putting their day off track. If I don't eat when I'm hungry, I become faint, anxious, and irritable. Basic self-care is tremendously important when going through a bout of mental illness. If you don't even establish a baseline for your body, anything will dip you below what it should be.

On that note, try your best to shower and wash your face when you are anxious/depressed/angry. Warm water can be soothing, and cold water can create a shock to your system and actually calm your breathing and heart rate.

In this piece, what was hard for me was I felt I literally couldn't do these things without feeling sick. If this is the case, talk to your therapist or doctor right away so they can prescribe something in the short term to help you reset your body like anti-nausea medication or something to help you sleep. You don't want to become reliant on these things of course, but if they can help get you back on track then definitely go for it.

Other things I can identify are my racing thoughts and my need to reframe. To help soothe racing thoughts, I've come to learn that a change of pace is what is needed to let your brain chew on something else for a while as you settle down. For example, forcing yourself to play a challenging video game or reading a book may slow your overloaded thought processing.

Something else I would do now is to reframe some of my thought patterns. For example, instead of placing all of the blame/responsibility to take care of the cats all on myself, try to remember that as Salem says, the best you can do is the "best you can do." Remember that my mom would say to just "zen it to the universe".

This is a helpful trick for lower level worries meaning some things need to be put out of your hands for the betterment of your health. In the case of the safety of my cats, I thought I was the only one in the whole world that could/would protect them, and I had to go to the extreme to do so even to the detriment of my health. This is not true. I could reframe my thoughts to say something like, I can do my due diligence and that's all I will do, and in the end, they wouldn't want me to suffer so badly to take care of them. The rest of my family has the duty of protecting them as well. I AM NOT A SUPERHERO. Being strung out to the extreme is also not sustainable, and I ended up going to a residential treatment center for OCD, where I couldn't be with my cats at all, theoretically putting them in more danger than if I was there.

Some advice for dealing with contamination obsessions in general would be:
- Zoom out! You are focused too much on the details and microscopic particles, when in reality, that is not how people view the world or how the world works!
- Most contaminants do not spread like wildfire. It is not like in the movies!
- There **is** such a thing as too much cleaning/ritualizing.
- The longest, and I mean LONGEST, hands need to be

washed is twenty seconds (not even necessarily in hot water). The usual time I wash my hands is five seconds in cold water. Every. Time.
- You can **never** be safe. No matter how many rituals you do or worry you put out into the world, so why bother doing any rituals at all?
- Chemicals and soaps you use to clean are probably more harmful than the contaminant you're worried about!
- If things have been safe up until you started ritualizing …? Hmm …
- Why isn't everyone as paranoid about this contaminant as you are? How do they stay safe without rituals? Hmm …

Cognitive Distortions to Reframe

- Catastrophizing – making something seem like a much bigger deal than it is (or minimization – making something seem like a much smaller deal than it is).
- Mind reading – thinking that you know what people are thinking or that you can tell the future.
- Jumping to conclusions – pretty self-explanatory.
- Emotional reasoning – designating feelings as facts. Ex: I feel like my hands are dirty so I must wash them for ten minutes.
- Labeling – assigning labels to others and yourself. Ex: I'm a failure (one I assign a lot).
- Overgeneralizing – seeing patterns when we have only witnessed a single event.
- Mental filter – only acknowledging one type of evidence. Ex: My ferret drank a lot of water so his kidneys must have something wrong with them.
- Black and white thinking – everything is either one way or another, there is no gray area.
- Should/must – saying that you should or must do something when in reality you don't technically *have* to do anything.
- Personalization – taking on too much responsibility and blame.

When Elenore Came Over

This next story is a continuation of what went on with the cats when I was struggling my hardest with OCD. In it, you can see the great lengths I went to to *feel* as though I had protected the cats. There are also lots of other cognitive distortions within the piece. Feel free to take a look and try to identify them.

I closely examine each piece of dirt and clump of dust and hairs I can see as I make my way slowly down the basement stairs. My heart jolts with each piece. Any one of them is a prime place for lily pollen to stick to Alice and Huckleberry's fur, which means they WILL lick the exact spot it touches and they WILL ingest it, and at that point, they are dead walking. I don't struggle to keep my eyes open, even though I've only had a few hours of sleep the last few days—my anxiety keeps my brain online and ready to jump at the slightest possibility of danger. I've never felt more awake actually.

My wet paper towel supply is getting low so I carefully walk away from the spots I've already cleaned and go get more while closing the door tight behind me, blocking Huck from exiting into the highly contaminated main floor. I'm in GO mode, feeling an almost twisted glee knowing that by doing all of these rituals, I will make the basement a safe—safer—safe-ish place for my beloved pets, and they can have more space than being cramped upstairs. I do not smile, however; it is false happiness, though I cannot see that at the time.

After spending hours upon hours cleaning just the stairs and the floor, something goes wrong, a small orange piece of what has to be a lily that I know was tracked downstairs is nowhere to be found. This means I'll have to vacuum the entire basement, change my socks a few times in the process, and when they aren't on, I'll have to wash my feet. But to do all that I'll have to step into the even more highly contaminated bathroom to get soap and water.

Hours tick by. There are times when I feel that I should

give up; let the cats die because I've done enough—so, so much for them, but then I picture their cute faces and their sweet dispositions, and I know I have a responsibility as an owner to their innocent lives. They depend on me, and I'm the only one who really knows and understands the danger they are in. Don't I owe it to them to do everything I can to keep them safe? Even at my own expense?

Suck in the dust, step, step again, wash my hands, empty their water. But I could have gotten pollen stuck on the bowl from cleaning so I have to empty it again and use soap and water. But I used too much soap and they'll get sick if they drink out of the bowl now so I have to take it back and wash it again because rinsing it is just not enough, but on the way back to put it down, pollen could have been kicked up by my walking and floated into the bowl, so it's not really safe. I vacuum more and more over the same spots, even using the suction hose on my cats and scaring them, making me feel even more awful, but I know that feeling bad for a few seconds is the better alternative to their lives being cut tragically short.

I go upstairs. That twisted joker-esque merry part of me is cheerful and proud of what I have accomplished. But it lasts as long as one heartbeat. I get a banana; I haven't eaten all day, but my stomach and throat scream in protest when I swallow it down. It feels wrong to eat now, when I could be doing more to save them. How can I just sit around and eat when I feel so strongly and ferociously worried about my babies?

I go downstairs one more time to do one last check. Then I notice something: there is a line of dust and dirt splayed across the carpet. Two lines, more. I feel the litter on my feet, and with a sinking feeling that almost causes me to kneel down, I realize the vacuum is in fact broken and I have been scattering all the dust and dirt and POLLEN that I sucked in around the basement floor. I see the tears before I feel them welling in my eyes, splatting on the contaminated biohazard of a carpet. I ball up my fists. I can feel my head pounding pounding pounding until I let out a roar of anger.

"Honey, what was that?" My mom calls from upstairs. I

start to feel sick again and then I am, as I rush upstairs and slam the door right in front of Alice's face, more worried about her ingesting the pollen than about her getting stuck in the door. That is the real danger here, of course.

I vomit into the trash can, ignoring her, before I call my friend Elenore out of the blue. We haven't spoken for a long time, but I know by this point my best friend Elle won't help me because she has already done so much and can't take the mental and emotional beat down that occurs when she has come to my house recently. Can't take how crazy I seem to her. And I know it's not her fault. So I call Elenore.

She is surprised to hear me at first, but as the tears stream down my face I get right to the point.

"There's an emergency with my cats. We need to take them to the vet or else they're going to die … and my mom doesn't want to spend the money but she doesn't understand!" Suddenly I see the situation through her eyes and feel, for a split second, I might be exaggerating, but I shove that feeling away just as fast as it came. I just sob and do that strained double inhale when you are trying to catch your breath while crying.

"Sure." She says coolly. "I can come over, don't even worry about it"

"Are you sure?" Knowing full well that I would ask even more of her and make sure she came no matter what, but I saw for a split second what this must seem like through her eyes and wanted to be polite.

"Sure, I'll head over there after I finish my shower, it'll be like twenty minutes. It's okay Casey." My heart tentatively leaps just a notch. If I have a safety person here, I can think more rationally and we can figure this out together.

When she comes over, I pretend she was just over to hang out and my mom was none the wiser to my schemes. I explain what the situation is; that the cats are in imminent danger and that we need to sneak them to the vet before it is too late. We spend what turns into a few hours in the basement. Elenore, having just walked into the situation and not knowing what to believe, takes a more skeptical approach to my worries but never makes me feel bad for having them. We examine the cats and research about lily poisoning and even call the vet more than once to ask questions about the situation. I am almost ready to leave the situation, as she had convinced me that even though there was a chance something could go wrong,

"I really think they are going to be fine Casey," she said in that calm, convincing voice. Until everything goes wrong.

I pick Huck up to examine his paws and he just splatters little drops of diarrhea all over my arm. I choke and my heart starts racing.

"I know that he's eaten it, he's going to die!" I am hysterical, crying and hitting my hands on the floor. "He'll die. He'll die. He'll die!"

At this moment, it seems like everything is pulled tight and while I'm losing it, the situation has yet to snap because I still have a chance at saving him. This rubberband existence has reality pulled tighter each time, stretching farther than before until I can't tell for the life of me when it will snap. I have a meltdown, crying and hitting the floor and walls repeatedly until a cut starts to form and the tears sting my sweaty bright red face. Right now there is no such thing as embarrassment.

Elenore wants to help me feel better in any way she can. She was and is, a good friend. We take both of the cats to the vet.

One of the worst things that a professional doctor or any type of authority figure can do is agree with you when you have an OCD worry. That's exactly what the vet and the nurse do when we go to BluePearl late that night just off the highway. The vet basically agrees that after the vacuum sucked up what I KNEW were lily pieces, that I had just spread all the pollen out all over the basement, and the cats had been walking in it so it was likely they were going to die from it.

She doesn't know, however, what I had actually sucked up which was probably honestly just dust and dirt. (Even writing this now feels wrong; there's a part of me screaming that I saved them; that there was lily pollen or imperceptible pieces of the deadly flower in that vacuum and scattered on that basement floor. There had to be. But it is with great humility and after lots of therapy that I can conclude that while there might have been, my rituals were for nothing and I was just a puppet attached to the twisted strings of a sadistic puppeteer: my OCD.)

The nurse agrees that I did the right thing and I feel valid for the first time in a long time. The nurse even pressures me further by saying that for some cats just by being close to lilies is enough to kill them. (You better believe THAT sent my OCD reeling with new ideas of how to keep them safe.)

They prick Huckleberry with needles, take his temperature, feel his guts, and keep him under observation. Alice is stuck in her cage for over an hour now. It's too tiny for her large body, and when I try to comfort her, she hisses at me accusingly.

Later when the vet brings him back in, I can tell by the look in Huck's eyes that he is terribly afraid and wants nothing more than to go home and rest.

All we had to do in that room was sit and talk in the cold darkness about all the money that I was going to be spending—the thousands of dollars that would come out of my dad's account after all this was through. The guilt hits me then, like stones flung at a sinner. My parents would hate me; they would simply not understand. They would yell or scream and it was all for nothing again because it turns out that Huck was okay this whole time. I cried a little when the vet came in. She is nothing if not confused. Hadn't I just found out that my pet was safe?

After we drive home, I know that even though they had been safe in the contaminated basement, I shouldn't take my chances. I decide the middle of the night was a good time to keep Elenore with me while I bring their food and litter boxes upstairs, and vacuum, though my mom was asleep. This takes another few hours. I have kept Elenore from eating for many hours and I definitely wasn't doing so hot myself. After she finally leaves, I honestly don't remember if I slept that night. How could I knowing that once they got the bill, the wrath of my parents would be upon me and the cats still weren't completely safe. If anything were to happen to them I would just die. I just would! I just would.

These situations with the cats describe the absolute worst my OCD has ever gotten in my entire life. There are so many mistakes I made and tactics I could have used to lessen my suffering, but I simply didn't have the tools yet at my disposal to do so.

As I look back on these occasions one thing stands out like a shock of electricity: *resist.* That one word can feel like such a burden, such a complete impossibility when you are in the thick of it that we tend to just succumb to the rituals over and over and over until all you have left are your bones. The main way you can learn to resist is to practice resisting. If you resist smaller compulsions that prey upon you successfully, then you can step up and resist even harder things until you have won your mind back. The key to resisting compulsions is *not* trying to avoid anxiety (this could mean distracting yourself, giving yourself reassurance as you stop a ritual, essentially not pushing through that anxiety) but to let yourself feel it wholeheartedly. *Sit with it.* Feel it. don't let a watered down version of your anxiety be what you win over (because that's cheating and not a real win that will help you any other time).

For example, when doing an exposure about challenging bad luck and superstitions, let's say walking under a ladder, don't cross your fingers to combat the anxiety of doing the exposure. That effectively is classified as "undoing" the exposure and that means you didn't do it right. Exposures suck. They are supposed to be challenging and uncomfortable and make you feel bad. By doing the exposure the right way, you will feel the anxiety of completing the challenge at full blast. You will respond by showing yourself you can sit through discomfort (not danger!). You will win. By essentially sitting down for a dinner date with OCD and allowing intrusive thoughts to come and anxiety to be there AND by resisting rituals, you have taken away OCD's power. Like the only way to get a tight seat belt to loosen, you must slowly pull along with it and it will end up clicking into place at the end.

CHAPTER FOUR

Journey Through Treatment Centers

OCD Residential

For some people, starting treatment may seem daunting, no matter the level of care. It was daunting to me once when I first went to see an outpatient therapist, but even though I didn't like him, he diagnosed me with OCD and led me to an intensive treatment center where my personal growth really took off. In different experiences I've had during treatment in the last six years, I've had all the way from amazing to terrible experiences. If you take away nothing else from this section, take away the fact that <u>ALL TREATMENT CENTERS AND THERAPISTS ARE DIFFERENT.</u> You can end up at a bad treatment facility or an amazing one. You can meet a horrendous therapist or one that vibes with you so intensely you feel you can bare your soul to them.

In my case, despite my bad experiences, I always knew that I was bettering myself in the best way possible through these programs. There were always people there for me during the bad and the good and everything in between, and I will be forever thankful to them.

My journey through one residential treatment center for OCD turned out to be the best decision I—excuse me, *others* made for me.

When I walked in the small back door to the building, my head was rushing; everything was rushed, like I uprooted my whole life and suddenly I was here. This long, winding place, forever. My dad dropped me off—I only got an hour to tour the place, set up my things, and say goodbye to him. I wouldn't see him or my other loved ones for at least a month.

My initial reaction to the place was that the people here seemed freer than the people who I had stayed with when I went to residential for depression. There was much more space to spread out in, and people moved and clustered as they pleased in the long, never-ending hallways.

I wasn't too afraid because this wasn't my first rodeo, and I basically knew how the treatment would work, as I had been through all of the different kinds many times before at PHP (partial hospitalization program). After going through my paperwork and talking to a few of the residents, the sense of entrapment began to settle in like a fog in my brain. I knew I would be here at least a few weeks—that still felt like forever. I still had the sense I would go back to PHP soon, that this would end up being too hardcore for me and everybody would realize I could just go back to partial treatment.

I ended up staying for two months.

The first day they mostly let me sleep (don't get used to that) because I hadn't met with anyone to make any treatment plans. The first night when I finally ventured out of my room to see what they had to eat in the cafeteria, I met these two girls, Reba and Max, and somehow, we all knew we were queer, so we instantly became inseparable. Luckily, pretty early on, I felt like I belonged. It wasn't just those two that gave me a place there, it was everybody—all of the residents. They just swept me up and took me in. We wound up being each other's biggest supporters even when the residential counselors couldn't bring someone down from a panic attack or lift up someone's spirits.

I started rigorous treatment the second day I was there. I was assigned a group, which we met in the mornings and evenings and relayed our bans and feelings (more on that later), and who we would do group treatment with. Mornings were definitely the hardest because we had to do a total of twenty timed chunks purposely making ourselves anxious in order to learn that we could get through it (exposures). While I had done hundreds of them at PHP, this was on a whole new level.

One of my fears was that I had a rare version of serotonin syndrome, which would eventually kill me. I was convinced on many occasions that I was dying right then and there. It's not like just a worry, it's *knowledge,* that you are going to die, and nobody around you believes you or gets you help. I would scream and pound the walls with my fists and cry my eyes out because I *knew* I was dying, and I'd never be able to see my family or pets or best friend again. So one of my exposures included having residential counselors come up to me at random times and telling me I had serotonin syndrome. I would have to stop whatever I was doing and start my timer, then only stop it when my anxiety decreased by half (on a scale of one to ten). Let's just say I had many health and death related exposures. And once you've faced death, it makes all of the other worries just a little bit easier to deal with.

Ban books also played a huge role in our treatment. Every day, we had to carry around these teeny little notebooks and a pen in our pockets or wear them as necklaces, in order to count our bans. Bans are basically rituals or compulsions that you and your team have identified to work on decreasing and eventually stopping. For example, some of my bans included, checking my pulse, asking the nurse questions, researching diseases and physical ailments online, and doing mental rituals like giving myself reassurance. Each time you give into one of these rituals, you mark down a little tally mark in your book, and the next morning you have to read off all of your numbers to your Behavioral Specialist and your group. Oh, did I mention if you don't meet certain goals each week, you are kicked out of the program? It seems harsh, but what else was truly motivating besides that?

We would spend the whole morning starting at eight working on purposely making ourselves anxious over and over and over (exposures). Then we would have lunch before moving on to group therapy in the afternoon. We would count bans throughout the day (even on outings!). The group therapy was much easier than morning exposures, but they weren't always rainbows and sunshine either. Some of the groups got heavy, or something from that morning or the night before was weighing on you, making going through what seemed like simple tasks horrendously difficult.

In art group one day, I almost didn't make it because I had been feeling lower than low and sobbing with my therapist. I showed up late with an ice pack to use a TIPP skill (ex: shocking your body into calm with the cold ice). I had been thinking about dying so much, the fear was so overwhelming and stabbed at my heart and took my breath away that I had become suicidal. It seems counterintuitive, doesn't it? To fear death so much and so intensely that you want to die? But I was so sick of the fear and the shattering pain of it all that I just wanted it to end. I felt horribly black in my soul and could barely speak when I got to that group.

But within that hour, something amazing happened. We were asked to draw, sculpt, or paint what we were feeling. I took black and grey thick colored pencils, and my heart beating sourly with cursed fire in my veins, I scribbled violently all over the paper, within the shape of a face. When I had finished, I felt satisfied with my drawing, my expression of misery. But then the group leader told us to rip it up. *Rip it up?* I thought with a pang of panic. *But I still feel this way!* Nevertheless, I tore it to pieces.

Then she told us to make something new with it. I didn't want to, but I must have had a drop of hope that day and I changed it, glued it, cut it, and colored it until I had a beautiful shimmering butterfly. I felt stunned at the accidentally found meaning. I can take my feelings today and transform them into something beautiful in the future. It may not be today, or tomorrow, but I can. I just did. One of the images in the set of tattoos I got a year later was a butterfly for that reason. After that, we had free time to ourselves and dinner, as we did every day (yes, even Saturdays and Sundays, we followed the same schedule).

Free time was a time to unpack the day with friends and to do a bit of self-care, like watching TV or playing a board game. I say unpack, not unwind with friends, because there was no real time off at residential. You were almost always in a state of turmoil of some sort, be it mood, or anxiety, even off the clock.

Of course, each day that went by felt like either an eternity, or a split second (anxiety will definitely make the time pass). But each day as I took on more and more work, got harder and longer exposures and new bans to track, I could feel myself growing, be it little by little. I was getting better. And at some point, I made a promise to myself that this would be it; this would be the one—the last residential I went to. I asked for more exposures every day to complete; I did my absolute very best on my bans. I put in my all, where at other times before, I would only give enough to make myself feel like I was making progress. I changed.

And then, it was January and I was talking to my therapist about discharge. I felt the stars in my eyes and my newfound strength beating in my heart when we chose the day, right before my birthday, that I could be free again. Not just free from the confines of that place, but freer in a way I hadn't been in a long time. Now, I would still have to go back to PHP before I could completely stop intensive treatment, but it was a massive step in the right direction. I went to bed that night smiling, knowing that when I woke up, I would be a day closer to that happiness I had striven for for so long, that had been snatched away from me that I knew I deserved.

Inpatient

Going inpatient was one of my worst experiences ... ever. However, I want to be clear right off the bat that NOT ALL INPATIENTS ARE THE SAME! While I had an absolutely wretched time at mine, my friends Sidney and Elenore both have happy and soothing memories from their times with others. My inpatient was in a small town away from my home, so they weren't very well funded. The food you got was the sort that you'd feel like homeless people would get at the end of the day when they were all out of the okay stuff. I only spent nine days in that inpatient (at my longest overnight residential stay, I stayed two months, but this definitely felt much, much longer).

There was hardly anything to do at my inpatient besides

coloring, doing puzzles, or talking to the wired old homeless lady that was going off of drugs or the immature bitchy man who decided to harass the female patients. I actually came up with a game to stave off that boredom: rolling up the familiar hospital socks into a ball and playing soccer and handball with them up and down and up and down and up and down and up and down and up and down the short hall of my wing. At least then I was actually DOING something physical to get out my restless energy. However, one man on shift basically told me to cut it out because I could "hurt someone." Bitch! It was a sock ball, how could it have hurt anyone?

I spent the whole of that time learning one thing and one thing only: stop self-harming. Inpatients are basically holding cells where you take a break from life in order to become more stable or less unstable, until you can seek out more care that has less restrictions because they are less worried about you hurting yourself. (We weren't allowed to have plastic knives, mirrors, or even pencils. We resorted to crayons.)

They had some groups attempt to teach us to lead more stable lives, but honestly like I said before, the only thing I actually got out of inpatient was that if I kept self-harming, there was going to be hell to pay; I'd be sent here again. There was hardly any space and definitely no personal space; most of us had to share rooms. I had to share a room with two people, one of which was a cranky old bitch who snored and had to wake up at the crack of dawn every morning to take her meds.

The one good thing about that awful place was they had a sensory room which you could request to go to and hang around in if you were feeling overstimulated. In my case, I went there because I was feeling understimulated, but I never let anyone in on that. They had big exercise balls with bumps, glowing lights, crinkly objects, and mats to roll on. They also had a soundboard where soothing sounds would play if you pressed the right button.

They misdiagnosed me there as having borderline personality disorder, or BPD. And the medicine they put me on was ROUGH. Like I said, They kept me there for nine days but that was actually longer than I had to be there-- my doctor didn't look at my blood work that would have let me go before he took a long weekend which forced me to remain in hell a while longer than most of my peers.

All in all, zero out of ten: would not recommend that specific inpatient. But like I said, there are some quality ones as my own friends have had some good experiences with them, so if you need to go to be safe, don't be dissuaded. Safety is priority. I'm glad that I was in residential care when I was suicidal even though I wished I was at home and able to see my friends because I got to live a good enough life that I actually enjoyed seeing them again. If I had only inpatient as an option, then I would have taken it. I'm not suicidal now, and I'm terrified at the thought of dying and losing everything I worked so hard for.

ER

I've had a few experiences with going to the ER for psych reasons. One was
when I was going through such a rough bout of OCD that I couldn't eat and was hallucinating. I also went once because I was so dehydrated from being depressed and not wanting to drink that my urine was red. ANOTHER was when I fainted from not eating or drinking because I was depressed.

The times I had to go to the ER for physical symptoms of dehydration were short and scary, to summarize. Not much happened there except getting some fluids into me through an IV and sitting there, still tired enough to practically pass out again in the hospital bed. Long story short, always make yourself eat and drink even when you don't feel like it. You'll feel worse if you don't. Things are much harder to do and your symptoms of whatever mental illness is ailing you will be much worse when you don't take care of body basics!

The other time I had to go to the ER because my OCD was so bad, I had been up many nights in a row worrying and doing mental and physical rituals, with little to no sleep during the days. I had actually become so constantly nauseous that I couldn't will myself to eat more than a few bites of food a day and threw up stomach bile consistently—I lost ten pounds in ten days. My time of crisis was brought to a head when my best friend Elle came over, and I couldn't take a step in my own house because I was shaking so hard and crying and was so worried about the health of my cats. Needless to say, she drove me to the hospital where I was so lost and exhausted that I couldn't even tell the man at the front desk why I was there myself.

    I stood at the desk scrunching my hands into fists and then unclenching them at an uneven pace. I felt like I couldn't breathe and my anxiety was like a white blank sheet covering my brain in blurry fluorescents. The White Room.

    Elle startled me as she spoke up and told the man why I was here. For the tiniest fraction of a second, I was worried the man would think I was pitiful, and then I realized I was so it was alright. I deserved pity at this point. I had been suffering so thoroughly and so much. I don't remember sitting down or going in to talk to the nurse, but I do remember getting my shiny white bracelet to match the anxiety in my head and chest. The room was one of the back corner rooms guarded by police officers and where your things are taken away and put in sealed bags so you can't hurt yourself with anything. And I think also in case you have to be moved to a different location after their social workers get a preliminary reading on you.

    I remember laying in the white bed, IV in my arm, looking up at the ceiling, somehow still, STILL going over in my head what I would have to do at home to clean up so that the cats wouldn't die because of me. Elle was sitting by the other wall of the small room in an uncomfortable looking chair, but I selfishly was just thanking whatever gods there were that she was there with me. I spoke with a few social workers and crisis counselors. They were all extremely sympathetic and made me feel as though I should cry. I felt so loved by them and Elle in that room, and later by my dad who sat next to me in the same chair.

    The only terrible and scarring thing to happen was a small, yet big, thing. I could hear one of the police officers sitting outside my room complaining about me. He complained that anxiety can't get that bad, and that I should never have been allowed to be admitted, and that *he* gets anxiety and has bipolar disorder, and yet, he can work. His voice is seared into my head saying over and over,

"*Anxiety*? Why would someone come here for *anxiety*? Everybody's got anxiety!" I was still in a state of fright over everything to stand up for myself and say something, but to this day, I wish that I would or someone would have. Did that man know how many consecutive hours I had been up? How I hadn't eaten and yet was vomiting every day? How many pounds I'd lost and that I was hearing things because I hadn't slept? Did he know how my brain was forcing me to do the same things over and over and over and over and over and over and over and over and over and over and over again to the point of silently crying and hitting myself and walls in frustration? How I was too scared to even get tired because I wouldn't be sharp enough to take care of my cats and my furry friends would die?

I wouldn't take my medicine that had a side effect of making me sleepy either. They practically forced me to take it at the hospital or I couldn't leave. They also made me eat. I think that was the best chicken noodle soup I'd ever had.

Partial Hospitalization and Intensive Outpatient Programs

Besides one of my residential experiences, PHP and IOP were definitely the most helpful in treating my OCD and depression. I had a variety of BSs or behavioral specialists there including John, Jim, and lastly, June. The one by far that had the most lasting impact on me, who I still see outpatient today, is June. She's the one who began the long, arduous process of rewiring my brain and taking me through rigorous training in order to beat the OCD. And I am forever grateful to her dedication and how she always pushed me to go above and beyond my comfort zone.

Partial programs are designed so you can still live and connect with the outside world while you do treatment. While

I was too exhausted everyday to have a job at the same time as program, I knew people who did. (Though I'm not sure how as when I would get home every day I would take a freakishly long nap because my brain was just exhausted beyond words.)

You would first arrive at a check in group where you would list your feelings, goals, and what homework you accomplished the night before. It started at eight a.m. so I was always really sleepy during it. Next, you would go in your assigned room and wait to see your behavioral specialist; mine, the majority of my stays, being June. We would plan the types of exposures I would do for the day as well as get anything urgent off of my chest. Then you would get to it. Work was hard and grueling—I did some of the hardest and most important work that I will do my entire life there in that little windowless room on the sixth floor.

There was a time where I cried every day. Things were so difficult at home and at program doing my work. But June and the art therapist, Ava, were always there for me, and would take time out of their days to cheer me up as my brain became a different organ altogether.

In the afternoons, we had a lunch break where I would go to the deli downstairs and talk to the nice lady at the register about my studies or whatever shirt I was wearing that day before eating. Sometimes I sat with friends, and other times I needed some space, but lunch was always a godsend from the heavens themselves.

Next we had group therapy which consisted of cognitive behavioral, dialectical behavioral, and acceptance and commitment therapies all on a rotation of lessons. I was actually admitted so often that I eventually helped to lead some sessions, which helped me solidify my core learning even more.

Overall, I'm so thankful to all of the hard working therapists and patients who helped make my stay bearable; at times, enjoyable, as I toiled away at rewiring my brain for the betterment of myself. There's nothing I would change about my experiences there.

<u>Second inpatient</u>
    Beautiful things can come out of horrible situations. That doesn't mean that anything "happens for a reason" or any of that bullshit. (I believe that there is no inherent meaning to the universe but simply that you can create your own meaning and that is how one lives a fulfilling life). While a person may be depressed, it doesn't mean they can't be happy too. And obviously, I'm not talking about one extreme of happiness, but instead, one can share happy moments with themselves or others even amidst the horror of the coil of depression. I once got out of an inpatient stay that lasted five long, arduous days because of a sudden drop in mood and forgetting to take my birth control. (Hormones or lack thereof can make a *huge* difference in your body!) It was the usual in certain ways: one long hallway, filled with broken and beaten people (and hopeful people too). Your rights are stripped away and you are forced to toil in boredom. But this stay was different from my previous stay in some ways as well: staff actually cared about me and provided comfort when truly needed. The facility was clean, bright, and filled with many INDIVIDUAL rooms, which are all things so desperately needed in times like these.
    I had violently wanted to die. It didn't matter how, the closest I got was to fill the bathtub and let myself sink into it. I almost took a deep breath, but aborted for some unknown reason. As I lay there, I wondered if that was what it felt like to be dead. I leapt out of the bath and slept in my mom's room that night seeking warmth of another, warmth that I couldn't give myself.
    But the beauty that came from my horrible experience; the beauty that shone through was inspired by my fellow jail mate who had two seriously deep scars still fresh on his arm. He wrote poetry, he wrote stories. Beauty came from this man who had tried to leave this world for good. His beauty prevailed and inspired me.
    This is the piece I wrote in my room, the sun shining through my blinds on the little wooden side table on the backs of the printed out mandalas my doctor so graciously provided me:

Twirling, floating drifting droplets of summer.

They fall like hot snow upon us; the sunlight dappled field we sit upon, faces framed by the soft breeze which carries them.

Laughter, yellow and bright like the light, drifts like a dream toward me.

It isn't quiet, but the crying of the cicadas rings so loudly with nostalgia that it is as if it is so.

My soul, like an unrippling pool, reflects the spotting of clouds and droplets against the blue sky, and I look up to see the endless spread of summer everlasting, existing in a rotation of seasons and yet all combining and stretching into one effortless moment.

Effortless, effortless sitting here, heart and body comfortably warm and face cool.

The tang of lemonade on our tongues and the hiss of some far off sprinkler.

A droplet of sunshine, a droplet of water now, and a happy cry of surprise as water bursts out from across the grass, the sprinklers having reached us.

We spring up, ready to dance in the spray as the summer wind droplets dance right along with us.

During that journey I met good but battered souls just like mine, each providing their own light even despite the darkness that threatened to overtake them. That was in the summer. Now it is November and I still wear a suicide prevention awareness bracelet 24/7 to remind me of my stay and of the people I met; of their trials and courage. And Mine too.

Starting ERP (Exposure and Response Prevention)

When starting ERP, there is only one way to look at it: like it's the most important thing you'll ever do for yourself. This is because it is. OCD is hell, but ERP literally can save you. Here I'll go into detail about how an exposure might be done, and how your reactions dictate the outcome of the therapy.

There are many many many different types of exposures that will be tailored to your specific needs. This is not to say that in treatment you don't treat all fears the same because you do: there is no special way to work on them because the content of the OCD is not what matters, it's the OCD itself. For example, I could have a fear of cats and another person could have a fear of accidentally hurting others. It may seem like these two fears are so totally different they need completely different strategies on how to get rid of them. Nope! (Also, ERP may not get rid of your fear, but it sure can make it easier to deal with!) In these cases, these people could both spend time around knives or cats in order to have their anxiety rise and fall like a bell curve over and over and over, until they habituate to the exposure.

This, of course, isn't what a therapist will have you do from the very beginning; as you can probably tell these are more high level exposures, and throwing someone into one at the very beginning won't help, it will trigger you into a possible panic attack. This controversial method is called flooding. Not to worry (about this anyway), your therapist will start you off with little exposures and as you build up tolerance or habituation to them, they will get increasingly difficult until you can truly face your fears head on. For example, with the fear of cats, your therapist may ask you to simply write the word "cat" over and over until your anxiety goes down for that specific run of the exposure. Usually, a good number to get it to go down to would be by half. So if you started out at a level ten anxiety writing the word cat, it should go down to five before you can say you really completed the exposure. While this is immensely challenging, it is for your own good, as without habituation to an exposure, there is no point of scaring yourself over and over.

On that note, now let's talk about the response part of ERP. As I said before, ERP stands for exposure response prevention, meaning that you cause exposure to a trigger, and then prevent your natural response, which would be a compulsion/ritual. Let's take the cat example a step up. Let's say you worked your way up to looking at pictures of cats online (yay you!), but after you look at them, your urge to ritualize by blinking twice hard is overwhelming. This point is crucial because the point is not to try and make the urge to ritualize go away and make it easier for you to avoid doing the ritual, but instead, you are supposed to sit with the urge, no matter the intensity, until you can resist through that intensity. Again folks, the point of ERP is not to make rituals and obsessions go away completely (they might some or by a lot!), but it is really like Jedi training in order to be able to live your life and not get tripped up by the hard things when they pop up.

Exposures are what saved me, but at the same time, they caused me lots of pain. It's so cheesy I can hardly write it, but no pain no gain. I pretty much cried every day when I first started doing them. Why? Because I was facing my fears! Things that I had bottled up and avoided with countless strange rituals until all I could hear was the screaming in my head, begging for a release. ERP is the hardest thing I've ever done, and one of the absolute most worthwhile. I definitely consider my ERP training for my brain that totally rewired it (with the help of meds of course), and I consider it a thousand times more important than literally anything I did in school. WIthout ERP, I may quite literally be dead due to the depressive spiral I went into because of my OCD. SO I'm just going to take the time, right now, to say, thank you ERP. Say it with me: THANK YOU ERP! YOU ARE A CHALLENGING MOTHERFUCKER BUT YOU ARE A SAVIOR AS WELL. The duality of man.

There are lots of different types of exposures that can be done, but I'll talk about some common ones and ones I did here:

- Worst case scenarios. This means taking the time to write out a story that builds with anxiety up until it reaches the worst possible ending for the thing you are worried about that you can imagine.
- Picture boards—making a presentation on Google Slides or on a posterboard with anxiety inducing images and words. You can look at the images and touch them and talk about them to family and friends as if you were giving a school presentation.
- Interoseptives these include anything that makes you feel like you're going to have a panic attack so you can get used to experiencing the symptoms. Ex: breathing through a straw or spinning in a chair.
- Saying to yourself that something *will* happen even if it probably won't. This stimulates the ultimate anxiety response and should only be used for more seasoned students of ERP.
- Writing eulogies for people you think will die.
- Dressing up in a silly/unkempt manner and going out in public.
- Eating food off of the floor or toilet or out of the trash.
- Defacing a bible.
- Going against superstitions.
- Purposely thinking disgusting, perverted, or bad thoughts.
- Touching butcher knives.
- Petting small animals while thinking gruesome thoughts.
- Touching fabric that you have an aversion to.

Restlessness

I never noticed it until recently, but I have an internal pendulum swinging constantly in my mind. Sometimes when I grow very still, I can feel it swinging inside me, reminding me I am never really resting. This doesn't mean I can never be at peace, however, it simply means I am alway *going*, always ticking.

I call restlessness the sensation that occurs when your soul is swinging back and forth out of sync with your body and/or mind. That feeling when you're just itching to do something, when you feel the agitation growing, and you start huffing and pacing like an animal that hasn't gotten enough exercise.

This restlessness, for me at least, can turn into anxiety quickly. One of the things I had to work on, and still have yet to finish working on, is sitting with boredom or uncomfortable emotions aside from anxiety. One person on Tumblr with ADHD posted that they did not just have regular boredom but "malicious boredom," which I resonate with 100 percent.

ADHD is notorious for affecting mood from high to low. A person can get a mood swing from zero to one hundred in the blink of an eye and have difficulty regulating any type of emotion. While I haven't been diagnosed with bipolar, some people mistake my abundance of happiness in my good moments as mania because it is just so unbridled and full. On the flip side of that, my anger pulses out in explosive rage that can't be contained. My sadness threatens to drown me. One thing I've been working on is impulse control. My therapist and I believe this will help tamper the anger outbursts as well as things like self-harm and risky behaviors. Always be sure to ask your doctor for medication recommendations to go in tandem with your therapy. These are two sides to a very valuable coin and can only work when done together—I believe that very strongly. I have tried many times, to no avail, to seek only one form of treatment without the other and I only came away with disastrous results.

I know many people with other mood disorders that agree

with me tenfold. For example, my mom has bipolar disorder. Only through medicine and therapy was there a chance for her true self to shine through, only when she found a balance between those two things did my mom miraculously return to me as her good old loveable self. I know people who don't have therapy but only take medication, and let's just say things didn't end up well for them. The key to rewiring your brain is hard work, dedication, and medication to give you that solid foundation you need for success.

Freeform on Fear

When the fear takes over, it's more than just your brain being hijacked, it's like the intensity of your emotions has been multiplied a thousandfold and all you have to hang onto is the familiarity and continuity of your own flesh and bones. Everything else seems like it has been ripped away or turned around so that you can't quite reach it, can't connect with it. When you are in emotional turmoil, you forget about the things that kept you grounded day to day, like family and your favorite TV shows and books—games you used to play. Your personality is nonexistent—you are just the fear.

It probably looks terrifying: the mask that we slip into when things go wrong. It's dripping with emotional blood and oozing with the pus of fear. It's riddled with lumps and wounds of whatever battle we are engrossed in. After doing rituals or feeling the flames of fear and anger scathe your back all day, it's a lot harder to keep from going berserk; to keep your emotional wounds from spilling over with blood, from your boils to burst open raw. Embarrassment is drowned out by the rage, the lightning flashing in your eyes and thunder on your tongue.

You lash out at objects, people, yourself. The sting of a blade feels more bearable than the ripping in your chest; the accusations hurled at loved ones covers up your pain with anger and flings it away from your beaten, shivering self.

But this does not really help you and once you're spent, the pain and the fear come back to twist their claws around your neck, choking you. You slip the mask back on because you don't pull out the problem emotions by the roots; you don't peel away the hold it has on your heart.

Once you do that, only then will you feel peace.

CHAPTER FIVE

A Dive Into Mood Disorders

Your heart feels icky, an inky black. Sludge has clogged and slowed its beat so that you always crave rest you don't need. Each day, a tight roll of red and black mess holds you back like when you try to push yourself up on the lane barrier in a swimming pool: you can sometimes get your head above water but you always get pulled back down.

Sinking, endless sinking. Some days it's like quicksand, others you just lie there in the black muck, vaguely, distantly waiting for someone to save you. Everything is a chore and you feel chained, enslaved by your *duty* to life and living. You wish you were a ghost: hollow and floating above your body; no longer echoing with hurt and struggling to go on.

But something keeps you going. Something. A flower, a song, a face. An outstretched hand and you don't yet have the strength to grab it, but you take comfort in knowing that it's there.

Some people describe depression as numbness. They are desperate to feel something, anything that will pull them from the depths of stillness. For me, it was constant emotional pain. In my chest, my stomach, my face. It held down my body, as if weights were tied to my core. I would try everything to get it out of me. Cutting, burning, scratching, *screaming*, hitting. And they would all feel good or on the edge of good for a lingering second ... and then it was gone, and I would feel worse than before. Spiraling, spiraling. And nothing seemed to be able to take it away.

Sometimes the days will feel longer than the nights, and you'll feel an aching sorrow mixed with something reddish black stuck like a giant thorn in your chest. No matter what you do, you won't be able to pull it loose. This may be cause for further upset, or you could just let it be as it is. The way I see it, when you dwell more on the things that make you sad, other things that aren't even related to the topic you're thinking about but that make you feel similar, tend to pop up. These are just more junk thoughts your depressed brain throws at you for you to stay upset and frozen in life. If, instead, you stay mindfully aware that these thoughts are just getting hurled at you and difficult feelings result, you can hop over them without getting stuck on them and without falling into a spiral.

For example, if you are lamenting how lonely you are and you start to feel low and unworthy and anxious on top of whatever else you may feel, the thought that you may never find love in life could pop up. You could either feel sorry for yourself about that and lump on heavier emotions, or you could recognize that that thought is just your brain making associations through your memories of feelings. In scenario one, you may start thinking about how you haven't slept with someone in months or years, and how much of a loser that makes you, and you end up in the bathroom with bright new cuts on your arm. Now you're full of pain and regret and you sorrowfully believe this makes you even more of a loser, and whenever you try to get away from the thought, the feelings stick around because of the reminder on your wrists. What you could do instead is just make a mental note (no OCD mental lists please) that you just had another thing hurled at you to think about before moving on. You can either stop and dwell on it and get sucked into a cycle of shame and sadness, or you can acknowledge it and move on. You might not be able to move on right away from the first thing you were stuck on, but at least things don't pile up when you stay mindful.

Depression hates company. A good way to get back at depression is to surround yourself with friends that truly care about you. I know it sounds cliche, but just spending quality time with someone who understands you can be endlessly helpful. When you hang out with people, just make sure you aren't spending the entire time venting or ruminating, because then you might as well not hang out with them at all. Friends can also be good tools for advice, but honestly your treatment team will really know what's the very best tactics for fighting depression. Even when sometimes it sounds funky or like something unbearably difficult to do, the suggested tactics of your team are going to be the absolute most helpful when living with depression.

Another thing that I find helpful is when you hang out with someone, make sure you are *doing* something. You can't feel any positive new feelings when you are just sitting around talking about how bad you feel, even if you feel as though you're "getting it out." Talking it out with friends can be therapeutic, but be careful not to fall into the trap of rumination. If you are actively doing something with someone, listening to new music, going for a walk, doing a craft, or even getting a change in scenery, you are more likely for your feelings to shift or the bad ones to lessen.

This doesn't always work though; you just might have a day where you're feeling so horrible that nothing seems to take you out of your misery. In this case, I'd recommend using a TIPP skill or something like it in order to jolt you out of the spiral you're in. It's jolts like these that can make all the difference when it comes to feeling better or even just slightly less shitty. My personal favorite TIPP skill (Temperature, Intense Exercise, Paced Breathing, and Paired Muscle Relaxation) is using cold water or ice on my hands, neck, and face. When I get upset and close to having a meltdown, I feel angry and frustrated and all around shitty and overwhelmed. When this happens, I tend to heat up; my face will redden and my knees will actually swell and get hives. Using ice or water as a TIPP skill in this instance is almost always at least somewhat effective because it causes physical changes in your body temperature. Cool is more associated with calm and heat with anger and upset, etc.

If ice isn't your thing or just isn't working in a specific instance, I would try a mindful activity like five-four-three-two-one. This is where you try to find a number of things in your environment that correspond to the number you've chosen. For example, you start with the easiest things to find, which would be through sight, then find four things you can hear, then touch, then smell, and so on until you've gotten through all of them. If I were to do this activity right now, I would say, "Okay, five things I see are, a Coke can, my computer, some ferret food, headphones, and my Iron Man foam fan." I would list them out loud as I count them off. I would make sure that I am breathing steadily as I do this, in through my nose and out through my mouth. Which brings us to our next technique, 3-3 or 4-4 breathing. I like to use this technique to center myself when I'm having a meltdown due to depressive thinking or an anxiety attack. This technique is really simple, but if done properly, very helpful. It may seem difficult during your tears and erratic breathing to get the hang of it, but the focus is half of what helps you while utilizing this tool.

To maximize the benefits of this technique, sit in a chair with your feet planted on the floor and your hands relaxed. You can close your eyes or keep them focused on a single thing in the room. It may help to have someone with you to do this, but there should be some sort of counting slowly throughout the breathing process. If you're going with 3-3, you should count out three seconds inhaling solely through your nose, then exhale counting three seconds through your mouth. You can try this for about ten minutes, or stop whenever you start to feel your mind and body slow again.

This breathing technique not only forces you to focus on one thing, it also physically prevents you from hyperventilating and causes your heart to slow down, cooling your amped-up feelings. You may feel physically tired after this, as you come down from your racing heartbeat, heated face, and spinning thoughts. It usually made me tired.

Tips for Dealing With Depression

- GET OUT OF BED!!!!!!
- BAs (behavioral activations) every day. This could mean doing value-based activities, fun things, or necessary chores that people do in order to stay activated. THESE CAN LIFT YOUR MOOD!
- Don't wait for motivation, action breeds motivation.
- Surround yourself with friends and loved ones.
- Not every day is going to be a good day. That's just life.
- Nothing changes without work and A+ effort.
- Some difficult and overwhelming days, if all you did was exist, you've won.
- Every day you decide to keep living, you have won.
- Some people will never understand what you are going through. Try to accept it.
- Make a schedule!!!
- Exercise for at least thirty minutes every day. (That could mean jumping jacks and walking folks.)
- Resist detrimental urges like self-harm and exploding with anger, you no doubt will regret it at some point even if not right away.
- Use TIPP skills. (Temperature, Intense Exercise, Paced Breathing, and Paired Muscle Relaxation.) This means grabbing an ice pack to startle your body into breathing regularly and slowing your heart rate, working out or doing yoga, 3-3 breathing, and muscle relaxation techniques—anything in your tool box.
- MAKE A DISTRESS PROTOCOL. This can be in the form of a list that lays out all of your skills to use when you are in distress. This way, you can have your toolbox handy in case things go sour, and you can't remember what your skills are off the top of your head.
- DON'T MISS THERAPY!
- Friends are not therapists!

- Do that value-based BA. Even when it's difficult for you mentally, it's good for your soul.
- Take the time to capture moments that make you feel alive/make you want to keep living. This could be in the form of art or even taking a picture or jotting a note down in your phone. It could save your life.
- Make a list of reasons to live! Be descriptive and as thorough as possible. Even if your list starts out small, remember, you can always add to it. Keep it somewhere accessible like on your phone or in your wallet or purse. You never know when you might need it.
- Your emotions are valid AND so are the emotions of those around you.
- Don't be ashamed of something that makes you happy. As long as it does not cause harm to anybody else or yourself, you are always valid, no matter what other people might think.
- WHEN YOU ARE DEPRESSED, DO NOT LISTEN TO DEPRESSING MUSIC. There's a difference between getting out the angst and wallowing. Find the line and draw it for you.
- Make a body checker sheet to check in with how you are feeling. Draw or print an outline of a body and use colored markers to draw where you feel your emotions. Have a list of questions ready: What am I feeling? Where am I feeling it? Is there anything I need? On a scale of one to ten, how depressed/distressed am I? Have a list of coping skills ready to use and circle a few you'd like to try. Come back to the body checker later and rate your levels.

The Bandaging

Depression doesn't just up and become cured one day, you have to live with it, and sadly on my journey, that led me to more self-harm. For anyone who doesn't understand self-harm, I think the best way I can explain it is that feelings suck. They suck immensely. They are confusing and overwhelming and they live all in your head and your heart, a place nobody can see, that not even you, yourself, can reach. Cutting makes your pain tangible, visible. It makes you feel like you're doing something about it, putting it out there in the physical world for everyone to see. It makes you feel less alone, less in emotional pain as the physical is now all you can focus on.

The only problem is that it's a big giant scam that your depression uses against you. Cutting, burning, etc. may give you that sense of relief for a single MOMENT. But at least in my case, everytime after I self-harm, I feel good for a second ... Then there it is: the meltdown. Some people think this is because you get an adrenaline rush as you harm yourself that gives you the extreme high, like an addiction. But that high can only be sustained for so long and then the black chunks begin to ooze in your chest and you feel black as ever.

i hang up the phone, my very bones shaking. *"The deepest i've ever cut."* Practically echoes back out of the receiver. My ears are still ringing and my vision goes black around the edges. Seconds feel like hours and eventually i can see more than experience, myself panting, gasping for breath.

Water drips onto the counter from my face and i suck in a strained breath, moving quickly to clean up the gory scene. Wanting both for you to see my pain and hear it but also wanting desperately to pull extra skin to cover the gashes i so readily carved into my wrist. To shield you from this forever.

The knife and counter are stained with my blood. It'll get onto the floor if i'm not careful. Katy is still in her room, better hurry. i refuse to share this with anyone else. I simply cannot share this with anyone but you. i run the blade under the water, smoothing over the edges with my thumb as my heartbeat pounds in my chest. What will she think of me when she sees this? i wonder with sick curiosity and fear. Touching the blade almost makes me want to cut one more time. A few more times. I feel sick. No, i think i never want to cut again.

    Two knocks on my door and a strained voice. i open it and you're there, calm pragmatic exterior, with a laughably large first aid kit. i lock us in the bathroom and start to cry.

    "i'm worried i might need stitches this time. i really messed up, didn't i?" You hold the back of my hand and gently examine my shame.

    "Well what matters is you stopped, right?"

    i sniffle and wipe my eyes.

    "I guess." i mutter, still feeling the swirling black clouds squeezing my chest, still trembling with the force of it.

    "We can always go to the doctor later if you need to, but I don't think this needs stitches."

    i frown before you can catch it, bite my tongue to keep from saying,

    'i wish more than anything that i did need them".

    You let me rub the ointment on my skin and it rages before it feels better, and I extend my arm out to you, needing this support, this comfort; needing someone to take care of me —needing you. You make a light almost-joke. You brighten my mood even just the tiniest of a fraction. Your steady voice keeps me sane through all of the stinging on my skin and the panging of my heart; there's light at the end of the tunnel of my swirling emotions. i can feel your touch, light, and caring on my arm as you help to apply the bandaids. i readily open myself to you. In this moment, i feel so extraordinarily vulnerable, bruised and beaten. Attacked, not by myself, but by life. Your touch feels so raw, so electric in this everlasting moment, and yet I never once think to pull away.

    You finish off by wrapping the bandages slowly around my arm, and my heart beats faster still. This moment forever suspended in the back of my mind will be over in real time soon, and your touch lingers as you withdraw your hands. My heart calls out, guilty for doing so that it's quiet, like a whispered scream. I hate being alone. *But you're not. You're so loved.* The last near silenced tattered piece of positivity inside me calls, and I thank you. I'll smile for you tomorrow.

If you self-harm for any reason, you are not alone. While it is not a helpful coping mechanism, it is one that many people use for one reason or another. It's something I struggle with to this day and has been one of the hardest habits to break. I think one of the most difficult things about it is the shame that surrounds it and the tendency to hide it.

One of the things that helps is talking about it to a therapist or someone you consider a trusted friend. I'm not saying you have to scream it from the rooftops that you do it, but hey, if you want to you can.

Another part of the shame may be hiding your scars. Now I'm not saying that you must have your scars visible at all times, but if you are in a safe environment, try letting them peek out. It's something you went through—battle scars. And if somebody doesn't like that then that's their problem. Free yourself from hot, overbearing sweatshirts and long sleeves in the summer.

Most importantly, find support from loved ones and someone trained in working with people who self-harm. The biggest thing to remember is that you CAN control your actions and you do not need to resort to self-harm each time you feel you're in crisis. If you can, find a reason not to self-harm. It doesn't have to be for yourself at first. It can be because you don't want your loved ones to go through the pain of seeing you do suffer. It can be so your arm or whatever body part is smooth and clear of blemishes. It can be because you don't *want* to. The last one may sound weird, but if you ever take a look at yourself in your best moments, try asking yourself: would you self-harm right now? Hopefully the answer is no, and you can write down a little note to yourself as a reminder that when you are in your right mind, you wouldn't do that to yourself so why should you now?

 Another technique to use is to imagine your favorite person or pet or even a celebrity—anyone you really love, wanting to self-harm. Would you want them to do it? If not, then why are you doing it to yourself? Everybody has, has had, or will have bonds. Why put yourself or other people through the pain of your self-harming? Of course, the goal is to find internal motivation not to self-harm eventually, but again, anything that stops you is where you can start. There is not one scar that I don't regret when I feel good later on.

A Dive Into Mood Disorders (cont.)

While this book has primarily been about OCD so far, I'd like to take some time to jump to the other main topic: mood disorders. For a lot of people, depression seems to come out of nowhere, just one day you wake up on the wrong side of the bed, only it's across the other side of the ocean, and from then on out, you feel it: that black blanket enveloping your soul, and that demonic veil over your eyes. But for other people, there is a trigger that starts a decline in mood, and no matter how happy a person you are naturally, that's shoved out of the way for less than tasteful feelings and thoughts. My personal decline into depression was due to the severity of my OCD. I have helminthophobia, which is the fear of contracting a parasite. My mom had the same fear, and after our puppy got one, we went into folie à deux and I became absolutely convinced that parasites had infiltrated my body and curled around my inner self. What could be more disgusting than that?

I ended up doing test after disgusting test (stool samples are required to diagnose them) and got a colonoscopy and an endoscopy and as each test came back with good news, I *still* didn't believe that I was fine. This is the nature of OCD. We will go to the ends of the earth to seek reassurance, and once we find it, it becomes useless.

Soon after I struggled with this fear, I went to treatment at a partial hospitalization program that handled my OCD well but didn't have the capacity to change my increasingly depressed mood. Imagine you believe you have parasites ravaging your body and nobody believes you. You feel disgusted and ashamed, scared to death that not only will you see them come out of you but that your carelessness will be responsible for you passing them on to someone else. I began self-harming. Disgusted and angry and afraid. That's when they sent me to residential treatment where I could be safe, even if only for a while ...

There is no substitute for when

your soul twists sour

   And your heart turns black.

The ringing of your ears
Almost convinces you

To stop

But the tears streaming
And the shower beating

Are not satisfied and the

Thump Thump Thumping

Grows louder

Until you see

Red.

Red behind your eyes.

Red noises in your head.

Red dripping down your arm.

All Screaming at you

To continue.

And so you

Cut

And slash

And tear

And scratch

Until the sting of the shower water

Is almost too much to bear

And your tears

Mix with

Your water

Your dirt

Your blood

Your pain

And wash

Down down down

The drain.

And then the fear sets in

And you're

Exhausted

Restless

Overflowing with shame and

Regret

And you dare to hope

That the bandages

Might this time conceal

Your most overwhelming feelings

And the red.

Reconciling With My Younger Self

Sometimes, the lowest of my lows stem from not only feeling badly about how I've acted towards other people, but also how I've treated myself. There was a time when I felt I had destroyed my body and brain and that my true self—my younger self was gone or hidden; traumatized by what I've done to them. After expressing this to my June, knowing I was a writer, she had me create this piece on reconciling with my younger self as an outlet for my shame and depression:

I blink. A sun streaked glow sweeps my face as I walk curiously around the edge of the park. My park, Tom Stone park —how it was ten years or so ago, with its almost-dangerous tube slide and purple climbing stacks. I wonder fleetingly if I am dreaming and decide that I'm not. The air smells faintly of summer-scorched wood and sand, and I close my eyes against a breeze that brings it towards me.

There are many children playing at the park, giggling and chasing each other, squealing on the swing set and bouncing their friends on the metal and rubber bridge mercilessly. I smile as I regard each of them until something, some feeling of nostalgia tugs at my heart, threatening to tear a piece off. The feeling tells me to turn around and I stop, turning towards the dangling bars and backtrack towards the swing set where a child in a blue and white striped t-shirt swings merrily while chatting away with their dark-haired friend who is watching them safely from the wood chips.

I feel more than hear their conversation, like background whispers in a song that you can't quite make every word out, but the feeling is there. I have that strange feeling again, along with the prickling anxiety in the bottom of my chest like something is off, like this is a dream.

Whatever it is fades away as the little kid jumps off the swing and lands with athletic ease in the wood chips by their friend.

"Wanna do it again?! Let's do it together!"

I grin at the game, like I used to play. It looks like fun. Then suddenly I blink, and the kid and their friend are gone, fizzled away in the heat of a summer day.

"Let's do it together!" The voice repeats.

I give a start as I snap my head down to follow the sound of the high-pitched voice, coming from right in front of me. The child has grabbed my hand and looks up at me with as much seriousness as a small child could muster. That *I* could muster. I was me and they were I and we are each other. They nod and lead me to the swings, trying to jump onto one a couple of times, slipping until I help them. I sit next to them.

The light blocks out most of the rest of our surroundings now, but I can still hear the other children laughing and running about. I am sitting, swinging lightly next to my younger self at my old park but somehow feel a surge of yellow calm spreading through my veins. Something else creeps through me like the crying of the cicadas nearby, but I ignore it for now in favor of the gentle yellow.

What do you even say to your younger self? Wait. I cover my left arm instinctively, wanting nothing more than to shield the child from even the slightest notion that someone would ever— could even think to—

"I may not have you but you have me. I come from you. Therefore, I know the me I became."

I suddenly want to cry, scream, and destroy this place.

"I'm—I'm so sorry. I'm so sorry that your life is ruined, that all that has happened happened, and that I've injured us in so many ways I'm so so so sorry that nothing turned out how we wanted it to. I'm sorry."

I begin to cry, hot tears made even hotter by the sun beating down on our faces. I sniff and look forward, unable to turn to look my younger self in the eye. But they now swing on a parallel swing set, vibrantly colored in contrast to mine, facing me, smiling patiently. I try to tear my shame-filled gaze away but find that I can't look anywhere but deep into the wide, innocent eyes of my younger self. Which I ruined. Ripped away. Was ripped away from us. I feel the overwhelming need to pour every possible explanation and apology I ever thought out at this moment into the eyes of the little kid —but they just pour right back into my own.

The cicadas' shrieking grows louder as I speak.

"I'm sorry I broke our own heart, I'm sorry that I let my stupid thoughts and selfishness get in the way of college and vacations, I'm sorry that I tore apart our familial ties—that I let it happen; that I let us get so bad as to go to a mental hospital and to physically and mentally wound ourself and to keep picking at it over and over. I'm sorry I didn't enjoy life more and that I didn't live life up till now to the fullest, that I was so so so mean to Alexa and mom and missed so many opportunities due to anxiety ... I'm so—"

Laughter rings out above the screaming of the cicadas, silencing their plaintive cries in confusion. I laugh at myself, tears pricking the corners of my younger eyes.

I stop fidgeting on the swing, stunned.

"Silly! Silly you, I *am* you. Remember? I have been along for this entire ride. I turned *into* you. Don't feel bad for hurting me, feel sad for us being hurt by others. Feel pride for all that we've accomplished. You didn't attack me with OCD, or lash out our anxiety or anything like that *on purpose*. In fact, you didn't attack me at all. We have only grown and experienced things together."

They pause their grin to narrow their eyes suspiciously at me.

"You *didn't* purposely make roadblocks like OCD and intrusive thoughts just to hurt me, did you?"

A lone cicada chirps loudly in the distance indignantly.

"No! No way! Of course not!"

The child grins, all traces of previous suspicion gone.

"Then you have nothing to be sorry for, silly!"

I gape at them, the hot sun growing cooler and the sounds of children coming back into the foreground. They shake their head at me as they point to my swing set.

"There's some paint there if you want to decorate it more, but look! It's already got a lot of pretty things on it."

I look back in surprise at the multitude of colorful, swirling designs on my swing set that I hadn't even noticed were there.

As I turn to thank them, they smile and shake their head at me. They've begun to fade away into the blue of the sky and the calm of the cicadas and the smell of the hot metal and wood.

"And hey, you're only hurting me by judging so much, dummy."

I blink.

Writing this really made me realize how okay it is to be hurt; to feel broken or defeated. Some people have the opposite problem of feeling as though their childhoods were traumatic or painful instead of or in addition to right now. You can write anything that bridges the gap between those times, whether it includes an apology to yourself or the two of you (child and now) joining together and saying 'fuck you' to the world. It's all up to you.

I do recommend it though as it has been what I come back to time and time again when I'm feeling shame, regret, or looking for forgiveness.

Mood Regulation

"You're a wildcard Casey, a wildcard." My dad recently said these words to me as we talked about how "erratic" I had been over last summer and how it not only affected me but my friends, family, and coworkers as well. They really stuck with me because a wildcard exemplifies exactly how I've been feeling and acting.

At this point, I'm not exactly sure if it's because of my ADHD, or that it's just a thing on its own, or from something else, but I feel emotions in *extremes*. That can be amazing and wonderful and terrific, or that can drop me down an endless well of sadness, OR it can burn me alive with anger.

When someone with mood regulation issues loves something, it can seem like that thing is all they think about, talk about. It's on their mind every waking moment. Love blossoms in your chest and swells so high it bursts forth and radiates out of every pore. You physically feel that love in your entire body.

Any emotion can seem to come out of nowhere. For example, someone says something that gets on your nerves, and you feel an explosion of sparks and flames dance across your eyes, you are one slipup away from screaming, hitting, or throwing something. For me, being angry literally feels like the emotion is too big for my body to contain and I feel trapped inside my own skin. I feel like I need to "get rid of it" as soon as possible and to do that the best way seems like screaming or hitting or throwing things. (Of course that only adds fuel to the fire).

A good example of how depression or mood regulation can be both good and bad; once, I was visiting my grandparents and cousins in Ohio, and we had some downtime so we all decided to watch a movie. At the time, I was highly, *highly* obsessed with *Captain America: Civil War*, mostly because I felt a strong connection to my favorite character: Tony Stark. The love I felt for this man was severe. And when I say love for him, I don't mean being *in* love with him, but actually *loving* him and his character arc of redemption, feeling his struggles with mental health (PTSD and anxiety, and arguably, scrupulosity OCD), and the other relatable qualities. He was, at that point, part of my salvation from depression; a source to tap life from. (And if this sounds extreme you clearly didn't read the above paragraphs).

Anyway, I suggested we watch the movie. I got everyone to sit down in the big family room in front of the TV, and I sat there, wide-eyed and happy to see it … while everyone else was talking. The movie began and my cousins were on their phones. My dad asked me questions because he didn't understand. Who was that purple guy? Why were they fighting each other? Let's watch something else. My sister got up to leave the room and somebody suggested we go out to eat. They stopped the movie. I was crushed. This character, this movie that I love, love, loved to an extreme, that I related to, that I wanted everybody to watch because it was my way of showing them a part of myself while I was severely depressed, was not of interest to them. I literally walked into the bathroom and cried, looking at my blurred reflection, trying to figure out why my own family didn't even care about me. I felt that depression pain growing like a black stone in my chest throughout dinner.

While that obviously sucked, I look back on that moment now with a shake of my head. Because I was so depressed the way I was experiencing things was amplified even more than they already are normally. If that happened today, (where I am correctly medicated and using skills and also just feeling a hell of a lot better in general), I would be offended, but I just can't see my heart breaking like it did then. Which made me realize something else: when you are stuck in a state or have mostly only experienced one way of having emotional reactions to things, it's extremely hard to see the other possibilities. Having been severely depressed and then being healthy afterwards, I can see what an overreaction that was. You can't exactly control your feelings, but it's nice to be able to reframe and see truly what other people mean by their actions instead of what your depression or unregulated mood assumes.

CHAPTER SIX

Level 10

When the taut feeling of buzzing pulls at your eyes
and chest and you can
no longer hear the traffic sounds
or birds chirping overhead,
Your heart goes into overdrive and
Oh,
there's the fear following
straight behind, blasted like a
rocket up through your stomach and chest.
Your brain sounds
the alarms, louder louder,
echoing off the walls of your skull
and pounding tight as a drum.
   How much more can
You
you
take until
you feel a crack? A crack
Forming just under your eye ready
For it all to spill spill
Out?
The love red fear
The solutions
The *urgency*
Of it all
Ready to fall

Like blood out
Of the cracks under your eyes
The fissures in your face
The chips in your chest
The slits in your wrists.
You're broken it
Seems;
Breaking each moment.
The never
Ending
All
Encompassing
Fear Shaking
You
Until
Your eyes Roll
In your skull
And you Fall
To the
Ground Hard
And Lie
I
N
A
Puddle Of Blood
But
God WoN'T
Let You
Die.
Despite
The
Blood
loss
The
Taut
buzzing

Ke
eps
YO
UA
W
A
K
e

This poem was designed to make the reader feel out of breath, which is what I sometimes feel when I get anxious. To some who haven't experienced this level of anxiety a lot, it may seem overdramatic, but I stand by it as it exactly encompasses how I feel during extreme anxiety and panic. A million people with an anxiety disorder like OCD could write a million different poems and they would all look very different in the details, but I believe that essentially the same themes would be there. I suggest using poetry (and writing prose) as a healthy outlet for when you feel anxious or angry or depressed. While at a level ten, you may not feel as though you can write, which is totally fine, but after you come down, you can write in order to work through it. You can also use writing as a way to calm yourself when you are getting to the mid level of stress or distress.

Dealing With "Gross" Rituals

One of the things that people don't really talk about is how gross or "far out" rituals and obsessions can get. I wanted to make this account as real as possible to help people who think they are alone in having this "disgusting trauma or pain" in their life. If something to you seems like it isn't real or valid pain because it's too "gross," (which was one of the words my therapist banned me from using) you are not alone, other people have felt this way as well. Feelings aren't facts. Meaning that just because you feel something to be a certain way doesn't necessarily make it so. Whatever your OCD journey has thrown at you, or you have done in terms of rituals, all adds up to this massively painful yet

VALID experience. There is no differentiation between "dirty" or contaminated pain and clean "pure" or "better" pain. Pain is just pain.

I'm not going to tell you that writing this section was easy because I've been through treatment, but it is definitely easier. While I still get intrusive thoughts and sensations and memories, I am not immediately put to a ten and overwhelmed. I think it is more important to get out what I have to say and let myself sit with the anxiety and feelings it brings up than to bottle it away.

I've held my own shit. Literally. I plunged my hand into the toilet, chased shit, and broke off pieces to inspect it for parasites or blood. I have actually done this as a ritual to get certainty about my health in these regards on more than one occasion. Afterwards, it feels like you're extremely contaminated, and there is an unsettling and painful reminder of the deed in the form of smell that lingers afterwards, no matter how long you've washed your hands and scrubbed. The fact that I put my hands and dug around in the toilet, however, does not make me a dirty person.

At one point, I would have liked more than anything not to have done that. I wish I could say I lived my entire life how most people do—without handling their own feces in a toilet. I really really do. Just thinking about it brings back traumatic memories of one of my first obsessions: fear of having/passing on a parasite, worst of all a tapeworm. I feel like worms are stuck in my throat and tangling me in handcuffs of fear. I physically feel sensations that make me want to cough, clean or rub my hands and shake the thoughts and memories away. But I refuse to do so for the betterment of my ongoing health. As a form of sitting with it, I write this having parasites fall out of my mouth and the smell of shit suffocating me (all in my mind of course).

Even now, I had the worry that after writing this that there will be blood in my stool as a sign of internal bleeding simply because I thought about it too much again. Maybe that will be the case and maybe it will not. Maybe writing this will kill me. Or maybe it won't.

Everyone with OCD will know the terrible twisted feeling

of performing an embarrassing ritual, whether it be in public or in private. The pull to do something that you never thought you'd ever do in your entire life like reaching into a toilet overwhelms you. You cry thinking that being immersed in the stink and the filth and just the basic action makes you a worse person, someone to be avoided, someone truly crazy. You think that this is something you can never recover from and something that will haunt you for the rest of your life. Well, it may pop up in your mind from time to time, and depending on how traumatic the thing was, it may very well haunt you, but it doesn't need to control you, and it definitely doesn't change who you are or how valid you are as a person. A quote by Brené Brown (mental health guru) fits in here quite nicely: "What we don't need in the midst of struggle is shame to be human."

I used to be tortured because of what my obsessions and fears made me do when I was at my worst. Getting shit stuck under your nails and dirtying someone else's sink was just one among several that still bother me from time to time. Another would be that I accidentally pinched and grabbed and washed and lint rolled my cats for hours on end in a tiny bathroom upstairs to "decontaminate them" from lily pollen.

Another one that nobody seems to talk about is how "dirty" your intrusive thoughts can get. I've had literal in-your-face or on-your-face images and smells and feelings of genitals of my own family; of children. I've felt like they are in my mouth or touching my body or worse, in contact with my own genitals. Sometimes a color will get stuck in my mind, like flesh color, and then I feel like it is touching me all over or in my brain, or suffocating me.

OCD is predictable in some ways, but entirely unpredictable in others. If you look to your values, you may have more of an idea of what topics your OCD will revolve around, but in terms of what rituals you perform, that can be totally up in the air. People do what makes sense to their own OCD's way of doing things. For example spitting may, to some people, feel comforting, while to others, this is an abominable contamination practice.

The point is everybody has something about their OCD

that they are ashamed about, and they shouldn't be. OCD's pull can drive you to do things you wouldn't dream of doing while you are healthy. It can make you think things that leave you in tears. While doing rituals is unhelpful overall to treating OCD, you shouldn't feel ashamed for being pushed to the brink. It's *not your fault*. On that note, things considered little hindrances or pet peeves or not even on the worry radar for some people become a person with OCD's whole life. There's no shame in that either. What you have is an illness with symptoms, just as someone with a cold gets a runny nose and a sore throat, we do rituals and get extreme anxiety sometimes. And it's nobody's fault; it's just how it is.

"Strange" Rituals

One of the reasons I'm writing this book is so I can show people that they are not alone in their suffering, and that seemingly obscure pieces of their OCD journey are more globally experienced than they think. When I read or hear about OCD, it always seems to be sugar coated or not very deeply delved into. It's like people want to medically describe the instance of a ritual or thought but it is always void of emotion. They never get down and dirty with the descriptions or examples of how far OCD can really take one's mind. People, myself included, are driven to perform endlessly embarrassing or unthinkable rituals and have a personal, intimate relationship with disturbing intrusive thoughts or worries, that seem to make them feel distanced from "normal" people. Well I'm here to tell you that while I haven't nearly experienced it all, I've been submerged in the same pool as we all have.

I have nasty, painful intrusive thoughts that still show up and wreck me to the core. Many times, when I'm around my emotional support animal, a ferret named Sirius, I see myself slamming the door on his head that he has wedged in the crack between the door and the wall. I hear and feel his skull crack, smell his blood. I feel myself holding his limp body in my hands as I sob, wishing him back but knowing that I will never be able to play with him again, that I am a cold-blooded murderer.

When someone says the word "shit," I am flooded with images and the sticky feeling of feces all over me. I feel it on my teeth and taste it on my tongue. The smell surrounds me. If this was me before treatment, I would retain these sensations and images for the next few minutes, maybe even the next few days or longer until I feel like I'm buried in poop and everything I interact with is contaminated by me because I fight it. I would struggle to talk to my friends as now happy memories are literally splattered in crap making them detestable because I'm constantly doing rituals in my head to erase all of it. Now however, I let myself feel this as the thoughts wash over me, and make sure not to fight it under any capacity. It still sucks that I have to become triggered in the first place, but it goes away much, much faster than if I tried to use rituals to erase the feelings and images.

Another nasty, highly uncomfortable thought that I have gotten used to is thinking of the most inappropriate genitals at inopportune times. I once had a sexual dream about a family member, which sent me into a frenzy. What did it mean? Was I in love with that person? Was I secretly some sick freak obsessed with incest? Well, on one hand, yes, I was now obsessing over and had rituals to cover my anxiety over incest, but on the other hand, I was by no means sick in some way. The thoughts were loud and crystal clear as images of touching family members. (What I learned later was that dreams don't mean anything BUT there is a theory that sleeping with a family member in a dream means you wish you could reconcile your differences and become closer according to my therapist.) It even stretched to children and strangers, then my friends. I thought nobody was safe from my rapey tendencies. But through therapy, I finally made the thoughts lessen significantly.

I now know how to deal with them. At first, purposely thinking the thoughts and feeling the bodily sensations having to do with the sexual images was extremely difficult and what I thought at the time was unbearable. I now know there is hardly such a thing as "unbearable." The only way it would be unbearable is if you literally, literally died as a response to feeling the difficult things. Something may seem unbearable, and you may vomit and cry and scream, but at the end of the day, you'll get through it. Afterwards, I spent time focusing on just allowing the thoughts to be there and wash over me, and to allow every gross feeling and shameful feeling come along with it.

Long story short, I used to imagine detailed sexual encounters with my family and even children and lose it everytime. It would ruin my day; I would have to do countless mental rituals in order to counter them which made my anxiety worse. But ever since going to treatment, I can now experience the thought and simply look at it for what it is: an unwanted intrusive thought. It can't harm me or anyone else around me, it is simply a thought. People are allowed to have any thoughts they want or don't want. It could be the worst thing imagined in your mind and still be okay because it's **JUST. A. THOUGHT.**

I could imagine clapping and whistling as I watch hitler raping Jesus in hell while piss spews out of their eyes and birds fly out of their nipples and can just keep walking, going about my day as if it were the normalest thing in the world to think. Because it is. And thoughts don't have real world consequences. You can imagine anything you want and take solace in the fact that even if it feels real and is horrendous–it's not really happening. People have weird thoughts all the time and even though some of us are more imaginative or suffer from more intrusive thoughts than others, they are still just thoughts. It doesn't actually say anything about who you are as a person or what you like or what you truly believe. I've known people who were highly religious who tell me they've had intrusive sexual thoughts about Jesus and the devil himself; it doesn't affect how faithful you are either. AS we learned in program over and over and over, THOUGHTS ARE JUST THOUGHTS.

Before I knew how to counter these and countless other thoughts, I would ritualize.

Some of the rituals I did include:
- eating my food a certain way because I couldn't take a bite until I had a "right thought"
- cutting my tongue on my retainer because it felt "right,"
- picking at my head until it bled and then some,
- shaking my head to clear it of "bad" thoughts,
- disinfecting my cats,
- disinfecting the house,
- going to the ER over ten times because I believed I was dying,
- spitting or wiping my mouth because I imagined worms in it,
- cutting myself because I deserved it for being a bad person and not warning everybody about imminent danger all day,
- calling the police multiple times over a chance encounter that turned out to not even be a real incident,
- grunting and imagining a "sacred" cow in order to purify "bad" thoughts,
- clicking my heels together three times in a row,
- wearing mismatching socks for good luck,
- using so much Clorox my hands burned,
- imagining my family in sexual scenarios to make sure I wasn't attracted to them
- feeling like I had to pretend my fingers were ice skating on top of my yogurt and saying a script before eating it,
- saying "toledo" in a high-pitched voice every time I saw the word written out,
- shaking a bottle of green liquid every night a certain way while thinking a "good thought" every night from second grade through high school
- tapping

And so, so many others.

I now do almost none of these and if I do, I try to catch

myself right away as it's happening and plan an exposure to keep up OCD maintenance.

Rituals/compulsions can look like mine, or like anything. They can seem strange to one person and totally resonate with someone else with OCD. More common ones include mental rituals, contamination prevention, checking, warning, wanting symmetry, wanting things "just right," superstitious rituals, asking reassurance, and scrupulosity surrounding religions or morals.

I had friends in treatment centers with a whole array of different compulsions. One of my friends, Reba, would pull at each of her arm hairs and pull them out by the root so hard that her arms would bleed. This was because she got the just right feeling from doing it, and it was an attempt to reduce her anxiety. Grace would repeatedly ask people and check herself for cold sores, as she had learned that the virus that causes them stays in your system forever after getting one even if it goes away and that terrified her.

My friend Thane wouldn't speak to anyone or even eat for days because he was so busy going over mental lists in his head in case he forgot something important which would badly impact a friend or family member. Krystal had relationship OCD and would repeatedly ask people if they thought she and her husband were truly meant to be together. It kept her up at night crying, and she got chest pain because it was so bad.

That's another thing. Having so much anxiety will do things to the body if gone along far enough unchecked. Having health OCD can make things even worse because when you focus on an area for hours on hours every single day, you will start to feel maladies in those areas. For example, my acquaintance Dan and I were focused on our hearts for a while. He actually went to the ER over thirty times in just a few months because he was so convinced that he was going to die of a heart attack or some other form of heart problem. We noticed the more we focused on our chest area, the more we felt and noticed even the slightest changes in that area. I, for example, began to feel sharp pain in my chest as well as my back and shoulders. I even felt it under my armpit which is exactly all signs of a heart attack. Upon frantically racing to the hospital, however, I found out that I had absolutely nothing wrong with me. My heartbeat was just a little fast because I was so anxious.

Another thing that happened to my body because of stress was that I got searing stomach pain that would stab so badly it went up to an eight out of ten on the pain scale, and it would keep me awake at night. I started shaking and twitching, feeling joint pain. I started getting burning tingling sensations and numbness on my face. I had memory problems. My eyesight changed and I would become dizzy or feel faint at random. At one time, I kept having the sensation of being sucked into the floor. Being in the thick muck of my OCD hell, I went against my treatment team's advice and got all of these things checked out. And do you know what all the doctors said?

"You have absolutely nothing wrong with you."

Which actually wasn't true. The thing I had wrong with me which was causing all of these ailments? Anxiety. It was being drilled into me by such intense anxiety for such a long time that I became physically ill and began experiencing all these symptoms and more.

The brain is far more powerful than we can even begin to imagine. I thought I knew I had all of these things wrong with me. In many cases, I thought I knew I would wake up dead the next day. Being soaked in such extreme anxiety for long or even short periods of time really changed you as a person. But not just physically. No, it changes you mentally as well. **YOUR OCD IS LYING TO YOU**. You may think you have stomach cancer because you have stomach pain because you think you have stomach cancer. OCD is a slippery serpent that lies and tries to get you to bite the apple. As for unusual bodily sensations, sometimes the thing to remember is: bodies are fucking weird. They may do things we don't recognize as normal even though they are, or they might do things we don't understand

Effects on the Brain

We already went into detail on how OCD can affect you physically, but let's take a look at what it can do to your mind, specifically how, overtime, OCD and anxiety rewire your thoughts. Having an anxious mindset to a small extent or in specific situations can benefit you positively. For example, worrying that your cousin may fall off his bike and reminding him to wear a helmet can offer good results; safety at a low price. But when anxiety gets to be so intense it shapes your every waking thought, you should start to rethink what your priorities and values really are and if you are adhering to them.

One of my values is to have fun. I want to squeeze the most fun I possibly can out of life, because to me, a life without fun isn't a life worth living. When I was in the thick of battle with my OCD, I was most definitely NOT having fun. Sometimes rarely and sometimes not at all. I'm lucky that I am now back to a place where my OCD only affects a small portion of my life, and I can have fun when the moment presents itself.

With OCD, your mind goes into overdrive and you are thrust into what I call the pinball machine. The ball is the trigger or initial thought getting shot into your mind, and each thing it bumps and clanks into is another perspective, or you are trying to "solve" the problem by doing rituals and overthinking. The paddles are essentially being too afraid to let go; you are the one keeping the thought in there no matter how badly you wish it would leave because, in reality, you are afraid of it leaving. You keep pushing the buttons to move the paddles because you feel as if something bad will happen if you don't examine every aspect of the fear.

When you are stuck in the pinball machine, there isn't much joy you can get out of a situation because all you can focus on is the worry or trigger. When you start to think of more things as threats, it wires your brain to be more susceptible to that type of thinking, which is why you need to work to rewire your brain during treatment.

The same goes for depression, especially. Depression sucked the life out of me. It made gatherings with friends painful and desperate. It made sad things or difficult things even harder to deal with. One time I missed when trying to kill a spider my friends were afraid of, so I started sobbing. I just felt that bad about failing absolutely anything. Not only do you miss out on fun, but you miss out on adhering to your values too. You become too preoccupied with rumination and avoidance in various forms, and pretty soon, you've noticed that you haven't spoken to friends in a week and you've been sleeping for almost three days straight.

If you insist on staying in the cycle of depression and refuse to go outside of your comfort zone in order to get better, you won't. No matter how much you think you can sleep it off, no matter how much you believe that you can out think it, it just won't get better. In fact, it is actually teaching your neural pathways to think more of that way, so you'll have a harder time getting out of it more and more.

All Under the Same Moon

Sometimes I look to the night sky filled with wonder, the shining moon reflecting in my eyes. And I think that every single person who has graced this earth has lived and died under this same moon. No matter what they looked like or sounded like, what they thought about or what actions they took to better or to wrong the people around them, they all existed under the same moon.

Someone, a mass murderer, brutally took the lives of a handful of people. He jammed a knife into the skull of one, gouged out another's eyes. The last plaintive thoughts of the victims were drowned out by their own screams. Another person lived a quiet peaceful life in the woods somewhere. She had a dog, a golden retriever. She cared for the wildlife around her and was said to invite strangers into her home who needed shelter from the winter cold. Another, a painter, was an alcoholic who suffered from mental illness and bled his feelings in large sweeping movements onto the blank canvases, his only companion a spider who would pay him a regular visit.

The moon watched these people day and night. But the moon, not having a soul or a heart or a mind, knew nothing of right and wrong, good and bad and so had no way in which to categorize these people. It just looked on with a cold exterior and glazed eyes. To the moon, each person was just a person. No matter what thoughts passed through their minds, what actions they took, what mistakes they made, they simply existed just like the moon.

A girl sliced her arm open with a razor. The moon watched as she moved to clean it up, her tears falling to the floor. A man imagined himself raping a horse and how it would feel on his way home after work. He cringed, berating himself for having a thought as disgusting as this. The moon watched, and felt nothing, for to the moon, people were just packages of flesh and bone with little brains. They went about their days and then they slept.

The moon rises each night without a feeling in its body as it watches over us. It is very wise. It knows that actions and thoughts don't have inherent meaning and there is simply no meaning to anything. It watches and watches with cool, calm uninterest.

What it doesn't know is that we humans have hearts and souls. We need meaning in order to survive and so we get it ourselves. We create meaning to fill our lives with joy and purpose. What it doesn't know is that through giving things meaning, we set ourselves up for pain and anger. Despair.

What we know is that we also allow ourselves to feel motivated and to find ways to express our souls. We paint smiles on the faces of our friends and splash teachings on ourselves. We create, we fulfill, we wish and want. We dazzle ourselves and each other.

All while the moon watches.

We all get intrusive thoughts. We all suffer. We all experience joy and love and hardships. The difference between us and the moon is that the moon doesn't assign meaning when we do. If we all thought a little bit more like the moon does, I think we'd all be in a better place ...

The Ferret

I realized something as I sit here writing this with a screwed up back that was caused by worry: why bother? As in, why bother worrying? I have lost weight, thrown up, gotten into severe pain as well as bad situations all because of worry. Last night, one of my ferrets, Sirius (like the star), made a weird sound a few times. Well, it wasn't even really a sound, it was more like a puff of air mixed with a tiny squeak. Because he had just gone on new medicines for his upset tummy, I came to the conclusion that he was going to throw up and that that was an emergency somehow.

One thing I've noticed about mood and mental illness in general is when something is off about you physically, it's harder to perform at your best. This is true of most things, but with mental illness, it can become dangerous. Last night I was especially tired for some reason, and so A. my anxiety was just overall worse on its own, and B. it was harder to reason with the OCD thoughts that appeared. Just like how when you're tired or sick or not feeling in tip-top shape, it's not a good idea to be driving, or to take a test—it's harder to live with mental illness. The only difference is many times you can choose to forgo participating in activities when you feel sick, for example. But it's around the clock work for dealing with a mental illness.

Last night at ten p.m., I started to forget that when I fiddled with my lip while I dialed the emergency vet number and asked my question about ferrets getting sick. I had done this song and dance thousands of times, and yet because I was tired, I forgot that getting reassurance wouldn't help quell my anxiety, and I would be stuck reviewing word by word what the vet said in my head afterwards, checking to make sure I didn't misinterpret her.

So, last night I stayed up a lot later than ten. And when I did finally fall asleep, I must have been curled into such a tight ball because of my anxiety that I stayed in that position the entire night only to wake up in the morning with a severely sore upper back, still wondering if when I went to go check on Sirius I would find him in a state of distress, or worse, laying there dead.

So I was, once again, reminded of a few things: that OCD is a round-the-clock job to manage, checking and reassurance seeking, no matter the excuse you have, is harmful, and that all of this could have been avoided if I had just sat with the thought: why bother worrying? Either way, the outcome of Sirius' health is the outcome, whether I worry or not. In my case, I would have worried myself into pain whether or not he got sick. Why should I worry at all if worrying doesn't change the outcome of the situation?

And I chuckle to myself writing this, because while this is good advice and of course can help to a certain extent (as logic can only go so far with OCD), it is easier said than done. OCD and other anxiety disorders rarely listen to logic, so don't feel too upset if your anxiety doesn't go away, right away with this technique. It's just something in a list of some things I took away from last night's episode.

Sexual Obsessions

One of the hardest topics to talk about that I especially felt was important to include in this book are sexual obsessions, precisely because I feel like they're never talked about. When it comes to sexual obsessions, I've felt some of the heaviest and thickest shame surrounding them. I have self-harmed because I was so disturbed and thoroughly disgusted by things that were out of my control, my brain's cruel way to punish me for all of my wrongdoings.

I like sex. You could say it's a big part of my life in some way or another. Remember when I said I react to things in extremes and have trouble with mood regulation? That happens when it comes to sexual responses too. I see someone hot—visceral response. Now that seems normal so far, right? Well, I've also noticed that sometimes when I see something cute like a little animal or a drawing, I also get a physical response.

This was just a little strange when I first started noticing it, but there was no harm in it, so I mostly let it pass. But then, as I mentioned before, I had a terribly intrusive incestual dream. From then on out, I got loud, intense, horrific sexually intrusive thoughts about anything and everything: sharp objects, family members, old people, evil people, religious figures, minors, animals—anything you could think of that would repulse me mentally, but for some reason, physically garner a response.

I spent hours and hours doing mental rituals, trying to purify my thoughts and checking that I wasn't a disgusting freak; that I wouldn't hurt anybody by accident or worse, on purpose. I spent many a night crying because I thought I wanted to sleep with Hitler or because I thought I would assault a child if I got too close to one. This bothered me so—and still bothers me, to the point where I'll get so frustrated I'll lash out when I feel like I just can't take it anymore. But recently, after lots and lots of therapy and introspection, I realized something. That sometimes when you really, really, reallyyy don't want something, or are opposed to something, in other words the more you fight something, not only the more intrusive thoughts you will get about it, but the more your body will wire itself to have the opposite reaction than you expect or want.

Remember when I said sometimes I would get turned on by cute things? What was really happening was I would get so happy (feel something so strongly) that my body thought it would warrant a physical reaction because it was so overpowering and akin to the strong feeling of being happy over liking someone in a sexual way. Add that to an even stronger hateful reaction towards let's say the thought of sleeping with Hitler and BAM! Your worst fear seems to become a self-fulfilling prophecy simply because you worried about it. Now whenever I look at a picture of someone I deem evil, my body produces an unwanted sexual response.

Now you may be asking, but what if for me, it means that I have this desire to be with the person I'm worried is too taboo to be with? Well that's okay too. Just like thoughts are just thoughts, feelings are just feelings. It would literally be okay if you agreed with these inclinations and feelings, as long as you didn't act on your impulses—harming the other person or yourself is where things become not okay anymore, and as we all know, the one thing you have control of in all of OCD and mental illness are your actions (as opposed to your thoughts and feelings). The important thing here is that you don't suddenly stop living by your morals and ideas randomly one day. You'll stay who you are and your intrusive (or not intrusive) thoughts of harm, be they sexual or not, won't just randomly take over your mind one day.

But what if they do? You say. Well, if that's the fear then what you need to do will be extremely hard. You need to sit with the possibility that technically you could be the one in a million person whose impulses and intrusive thoughts will hijack their brain and cause you to harm someone. In my case, I could spend time with children, or watch shows on the Disney channel. If that's too much at first, then maybe I could picture a child in my life and sit with the anxiety that surrounds the sexual or harm response until it rises and falls, and I am ready to move onto something more challenging.

I did this with violent harm thoughts in intensive treatment one day. My BS basically sat me down and handed me a wide variety of sharp knives, and then sat in front of me with her back turned to me, totally vulnerable. She said, say aloud what you're envisioning and move the knife. If that doesn't sound scary enough, here was the big catch: I had been instructed to take my Ativan, which gets me high (inebriated and more impulsive), before this session. Even while medicated, I still felt anxiety creep over me slowly, pulsing through the haze in the front of my brain.

High with medication, fear, power, and disgust, I let the bloodied images and sensations that came with my intrusive thoughts drip over me as I moved the knife slowly from one part of her body to the next. My vision swelled with red, I felt the jerking movements of my hand and her body as I plunged the knife into her shoulders, her back. As I slit her throat slowly and let her blood spill over us, bonded in death, I felt twisted in my chest, my brain telling me I wanted one thing and my heart screaming with a fiery fury against it as it beat hard and slow against my ribs. I blinked and withdrew my knife, feeling like I had just poured out a heavy pus-filled tumor on my soul, and she smiled at me and nodded.

"See? You didn't do it."

CHAPTER SEVEN

Anger

    I have intermittent explosive disorder. This means that I get irritable very easily, and I can go from zero to one hundred faster than the blink of an eye. My chest pours out hot lava and my brain gets foggy so much that when I'm in the thick of a tantrum or a fight, I feel as though I'm not thinking at all, that my mind is blank. It's not the same as the White Room, it's just blank. Nothingness. My screams echo throughout the house as I become more frantic, insults flying out of my mouth hurled at the ones I care about most. My fists are clenched, my body shaking wildly. Blurry. The world is blurry. My head pounds and blood rushes as I feel strength akin to the nine-tailed demon fox from *Naruto* pulse through my veins and I smack the wall, bruising my hand. I truly feel like an animal.

    And I don't stop. Not when I break the bookstand. Not when I crush the metal garbage can. Not when my mom stands there and looks at me with utter fear in her eyes as tears drip down her face. No. I only stop when I catch a glimpse of myself in the mirror and like something out of a dream. I don't, can't recognize myself. It shocks me to attention, like an army sergeant has just scolded me, and I metaphorically dust myself off and try to reboot my brain so that higher thinking comes back online. I stare and quickly look away. I feel like Wanda from *Doctor Strange in the Multiverse of Madness*. Starting with the best intentions, I see what I've become. A monster, she realizes as her children cower in fear. The sour truth sinks slowly down in my gut: I have become one as well. I have hurt people. I've hit my mom who has shown me nothing but love my entire life. I destroyed personal property; made my loved ones cry and shudder in fear. That's what I am: the nine-tailed fox. I'm a monster, a demon.

    blurred droplets of
    red scattered across
    the landscape.
    hide away from pain
    burning bright
    the sting of tears of the claws
    in your thigh
    against me
    against me
    against me
    the whole world has conspired
    and dripped it into this moment
    into you
    and i rage.
    severing bonds
    severing skin
    black smoke pours out of my mouth and tastes wicked on my tongue
    but i
    i
    twist on
    bringing the waves up beside me
    redred upup
    fire
    and heat
    and everyone around me inhales the smoke
    but i don't
    CARE
    they did this to me
    YOU did this to me
    and im

> bl
> eed
> ing
> underneath the flames
> they burn
> so that i can rage

While this is how it can feel for many people with trouble regulating their anger, I feel the extremeness all around appears in how people have trouble regulating other "negative" emotions as well. And just because you feel like a monster, doesn't mean you are one. That doesn't mean, however, that you shouldn't step back and take a look at yourself when you feel an emotion that is as extreme as the situation above. I may have only just begun my journey on working on anger management, but I know some tips and tricks that can help with rage.

The number one problem that people with anger issues AND self-harm issues, as well as mania, etc., is impulse control. I know this because I took the time to identify it with my therapist, and because it has been pointed out to me on many occasions. Like I said, I'm still learning, but the way I figure it works is just like doing ERP for anxiety. Resisting rituals isn't that much different from resisting impulses. Rituals are basically impulses when you think about it. They're compulsive, that's why they are also called compulsions.

One thing I already know is that the one thing people have complete 100 percent control over are their actions. Not their thoughts, or feelings, but their actions. Even though at times it may seem that in something like an angry outburst or emotional crisis, we just explode, every way we react to those feelings is in our control. I'm not saying that means it's easy to not give in to impulses (believe me I've got a lot of work ahead of me), but it is 100 percent possible for you to change your actions and become a better, healthier person as you connect to those around you.

One technique I use is making a list of reasons why I want to live when I am feeling happy, so I can look back on it in a moment of severe suicidal ideation and so I dont impulsively end my life just because im feeling a certain way.

Another technique I just started to use is writing down all the reasons I don't want to throw a tantrum or break and hit things, as well as the consequences of those actions. This is a note on my phone I have readily available for daily use. If I feel I'm going to explode, I can simply look at the note and use that in tandem with a TIPP skill like 4-4 breathing and help me calm down, to resist the negative impulses.

That's the thing with impulses, they're always forged out of an overwhelming sensation or feeling. With OCD rituals, it feels necessary to survive. With self-harm it feels like the only way to end emotional pain. And with anger it feels like the only way to rise above anxiety and "get your emotions out." The thing is, the negative impulse is always the easy way out—the cheap plan that ends up falling apart in the end. What I believe and what I think I'll come to learn is that by not surrendering to your impulses and instead reminding yourself that you are always in control of your actions, you have taken the first step in winning them over and leading a healthier life.

You Mustn't Die by Your Own Hand

Some days you will just feel like shit. And sometimes there is nothing you can do about that. But this, however, is okay, because you have to keep in mind that feelings pass, things change, and nothing ever remains the same for long. You may want to kill yourself one day and have a great time at a party the next and that's so scary because what if you had decided to end it the day before? You would have never experienced this beauty, this joy, this LIFE that fills your lungs and sparks your heart to life. What I'm saying is, don't trust your urge to kill yourself. Your brain gets tangled up and then somehow latches onto the idea that it's a good one, and that it's the only option, but it's not. And once you learn that, you'll realize you are giving yourself a whole world of possibilities for love, laughter, amazement, anger, boredom, joy, and the whole array of emotions that make up the human experience.

Last summer I thought that I wanted death. But so many things have changed since then and I am in a totally unexpected and much better place. I have new friends, I'm back at school, I had relationships, I have a new second ferret named Koda who I love to the core. I'm back on track with my life and I'm happy once again. I look back on that dark time when I craved my death and I'm filled with intense fear. For what if I had done it? I wouldn't have gotten the chance to step into the light once again and feel the crisp chill of November, wouldn't have gotten to feel the softness of a new lover. Do your future self a favor, don't die by your own hand.

The Role of Imagination

One thing I don't agree with experts on when it comes to OCD is the idea that we all get intrusive thoughts to the same degree, we just latch onto them more than mentally healthy people. Of all the people with OCD that I've met, I see the frequency of these intrusive thoughts skyrocket at the worst points in our OCD. There is also another thing I have noticed: most of us seem to have overactive imaginations. And by overactive, I mean at one point, I could be sitting there staring off into space when in my mind's eyes, I'm lighting my fingers on fire and cradling the face of a baby, burning it and then suddenly I'm touching its genitals and the baby starts crying. I can smell the smoke and hear the screams and then suddenly the baby gives birth to a bunch of tapeworms and they surround me, strip me of my clothes and rape me. At this point I'm tied up, crying and I can't see straight but I can smell the acidic death coming off of them and then—my attention is diverted back to reality when I snap my head up—someone says my name.

But these thoughts don't just go away, the pressure from the tied-up worms scratches the back of your mind, your groin moves with the thought of a sexual encounter, you can still smell the smoke. And the emotions that come with these intrusive thoughts. Oh boy. The sadness, and fear and disgust that envelops you until it's all too much and you run out of the room crying, in unbridled fear for what a bad person you must be to imagine these things and to have this response.

Well I'm here to tell you that while I'm not sure this is normal for mentally healthy people, it is totally normal for people with OCD and *especially* those with overactive imaginations like mine. The truth is while many people experience this, nobody likes to talk about it with anyone, some not even with their therapist. And this causes a problem because then nobody knows that it is NORMAL TO HAVE "CRAZY," VISCERAL INTRUSIVE THOUGHTS.

Some people just experience them more than others. There's nothing wrong or dirty about having them. Thoughts, while they can be distressing and extremely annoying and upsetting, are just that: thoughts. They say nothing about a person's character, or worth, or level of kindness, or anything like that. Sometimes our brains just like to shock us to see what will happen. What you have to do in response is to let those thoughts come and to thank your brain for providing a new way of looking at something. And I bet most of us are pretty creatively imaginative as well. To have so much creative imagination power comes with a cost, that being crazy intrusive thoughts, but hey it's alright. It really, truly is.

Conclusion

I hope that what you've gained from this book is something that you were looking for, whether it be basic information on OCD and mood disorders or some advice. Maybe you were looking for more people who had visited the White Room and wanted to feel less alone. I hope you do now. The main thing I'd like you to take away from this book is that all people have funky and nuanced ways that their brains look at and react to things. Each brain is unique, so while we can find solace in our mental similarities, we can acknowledge our differences as well.

After my stay at the OCD residential, I got a tattoo to signify my strength and accomplishments. An infinity sign, a star for dreams, a paw print for moving forward, a pendulum for having to go hard one way in order to make progress back towards the middle, and most importantly, a butterfly signifying transformation and change. This way, I'll always have a reminder for my accomplishments glued to my body. They have become one with me. My journey is far from over, but I have passed the point where I have gathered the majority of the tools that I need in order to succeed.

My strange brain thought a tattoo would be beneficial, and it was right.

In terms of what you have control over, you can spend days and months and weeks and years regretting and agonizing over why you spent that time ritualizing or why you had an angry outburst at your mom or why you feel like a failure. But the key thing I've learned for dealing with these thoughts is this: the past is the past. We can't do anything about it. But the future has yet to be written. YOU shape your future through your actions and reactions. What better can you do after realizing you don't like the self you are or regret some of the things that you've done than try your best for now on to become your best shining self? And I'm not saying it's a straight shot to living your best life: people make mistakes. People relapse. Shit happens. But it is always in your control how you act and react and that's how you'll change yourself for the better.

The strive for happiness is a noble one, but remember that you might not reach a state where you're elated all the time. It's more like striving for a balanced life of highs and lows that aren't too extreme with you existing around a baseline of contentment that you should be more focused on looking for. This is where most of the neurotypical people sit from day to day. If you can find a way to have high levels of happiness every day, that's great (as long as it's not from mania!).

Brains are weird enough that as the days and weeks and months go on, finding something akin to happiness/contentment with life may be difficult. It is our job to work with our brains and not against them to find that place that we want to be. It is up to us to burst out of that White Room, crooked compasses by our sides and say let's move forward anyway; to look at the shadows over our depressed brains and jump up to open the window and let in the light.

Utilizing tools that you have collected during time in treatment can help immensely with bursting out of that room, or making the strength to get up out of bed when you are drenched in the dark ink that is depression. It's the little things, the maintenance things, that we collect and have to build up in order to be successful, but in times of crisis of course it's appropriate to bust out the big guns.

While this can be overwhelming and difficult, we have a duty to our future mentally healthy selves, as well as our current selves, to take care as much as possible. This is done for our betterment and the betterment of those around us. Our goals, our dreams, and our lives are all shimmering beautiful things, even with the rough patches that we enter. We should take better care of ourselves in order to keep that light burning bright.

Whether it's OCD, depression, or something else entirely it's important to keep in mind that we should push ourselves towards betterment while also not overdoing it. Because like it was stated before: the best we can do is the best we can do. Jump towards greatness; you'll get there. Even if it takes a long time, if you put in the work and the heart, you'll make it. You'll make it. You'll make it.

ABOUT THE AUTHOR

Casey Birchman

Casey is a 24 year old undergrad student at the University of Illinois at Urbana-Champiagn studying East Asian Languages and Cultures and minoring in Teaching ESL. They have a long history with mental illness and health as they suffer from OCD, depression, Intermittent Explosive Disorder, and ADHD. They wrote this book so that people could gain insight into their disorders, and so that loved ones could learn about these debilitating illnesses. Their dream is to help people feel less alone and more empowered in their struggles.

www.ingramcontent.com/pod-product-compliance
Lightning Source LLC
Chambersburg PA
CBHW071419210526
45465CB00001B/458